CANCER, MY LOVE

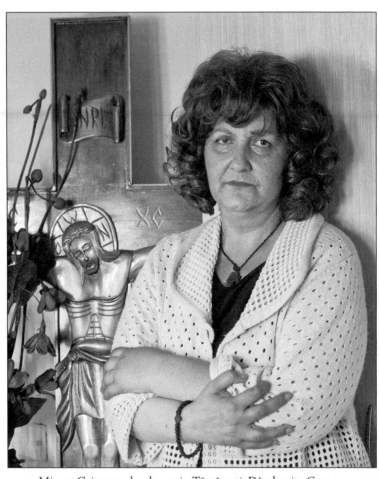

Mioara Grigore at her home in Tărtășești, Dâmbovița County, Romania, April 9, 2014. Photo by Dinu Lazăr.

Cancer, My Love

by Mioara Grigore

Translated from the Romanian by Oana Michael
and Simona Irime

Edited by the St. Herman of Alaska Brotherhood

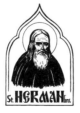

ST. HERMAN OF ALASKA BROTHERHOOD
2018

St. Herman of Alaska Brotherhood
P. O. Box 70, Platina, California 96076 U.S.A.
website: www.sainthermanmonastery.com
email: stherman@stherman.com

Copyright © 2018 by the St. Herman of Alaska Brotherhood.

All rights reserved.

First edition: 2018. Printed in the United States of America.

Translated with permission from Mioara Grigore, *Cancerul, dragostea mea* [Cancer, my love] (Bucharest: Predanie, 2014).

Front cover: Caraiman Heroes' Cross Monument at sunrise in the Bucegi Mountains, Southern Carpathians, Romania. Photo by Janos Gaspar, 123RF photos.

Back cover: Mioara Grigore (*top*); the Grigore family (*bottom*), April 9, 2014. Photos by Dinu Lazăr.

Publishers Cataloging in Publication

Names: Grigore, Mioara, author. | Michael, Oana, translator. | Irime, Simona, translator. | Saint Herman of Alaska Brotherhood, editor.
Title: Cancer, my love / by Mioara Grigore ; translated from the Romanian by Oana Michael and Simona Irime ; edited by the St. Herman of Alaska Brotherhood.
Other titles: Cancerul, dragostea mea. English.
Description: First edition. | Platina, California : St. Herman of Alaska Brotherhood, 2018.
Identifiers: ISBN: 978-1-887904-59-9 | LCCN: 2018932732
Subjects: LCSH: Grigore, Mioara. | Cancer patients' writings. | Cancer—Patients—Religious aspects—Orthodox Eastern Church. | Spiritual formation—Orthodox Eastern Church. | Spiritual life—Orthodox Eastern Church. | Families—Religious aspects—Orthodox Eastern Church. | Marriage—Religious aspects—Orthodox Eastern Church. | Love—Religious aspects—Orthodox Eastern Church. | Suffering—Religious aspects—Orthodox Eastern Church. | Mothers of children with disabilities—Religious aspects—Orthodox Eastern Church. | Down syndrome—Patients—Family relationships. | Biserica Ortodoxă Română—Biography. | Orthodox Eastern Church—Romania—Biography.
Classification: LCC: RC279.6.G75 G7513 2018 | DDC: 362.19699/40092—dc23

Contents

Editor's Preface 9
Foreword: About All Sorts of Gravitational Forces
   by Anca Stanciu. 13
Romanian Pronunciation Guide 17
  1. The Fall 19
  2. Stairs. 23
  3. Sicilian Defense. 29
  4. The Pilgrimage. 33
  5. The Fainting Spell. 39
  6. The Spiritual Father. 41
  7. The Wedding. 44
  8. The Wedding Night. 48
  9. The Birth of the First Child—Gray-Eyed Maria 52
10. Holy Baptism. 58
11. Anthony—The Birth of the Second Child 61
12. About Nektarios. 65
13. Anthony's Dilemma. 71

CONTENTS

14. About Macrina 73
15. Justina, the One with Dimples. 77
16. The Supremacy of the Lump. 79
17. The Defeat of the Tumor's Guardian. 83
18. The Shot. 86
19. Ruthless Malignant Cells 89
20. The Futility of an Explanation. 93
21. Death- and Life-Giving Chemo 97
22. Life-Saving Biochemistry 101
23. The Removal 105
24. The Flight. 109
25. The MD2 Accelerator 113
26. The Irradiation of Yesterday, Today, and Tomorrow. . 118
27. Wonderful Times 120
28. Meeting Supreme Joy 124
29. Egret and Her Wonderful Pills 133
30. The Big Questions of My Life 136
31. The Return 138
32. Aida and Her Notary Documents. 143
33. The Plumber and His "Living" Word. 148
34. Plescoi Sausages 151

CONTENTS

35. Nights with Stories and Water in My Lungs 159

36. Suleiman the Magnificent of Romania. 171

37. The One Who Saw It So Well. 174

38. The Doctor's Eyelashes 178

39. The Courage of Youth in the Face of Death 182

40. My Tears and "Ovid's Tears". 187

41. The Architecture of Sacrifice 190

42. Disabled from Yesterday to Forever. 192

43. From Vienna to Bucharest 195

44. The Long Way of Innocence. 199

45. Mesopotamia Not Forgotten. 204

46. Somewhere between a Broken Heart and the Majesty of a Mountain 207

Epilogue

1. Mioara, My Love *by Anca Stanciu* 219

2. "Mioara Gave Me the Chance of Sanctification through Her Life" *An Interview with Viorel Grigore* 225

3. "The Testimony of a Shared Love" *An Interview with Fr. Georgian Păunoiu*. 229

4. Message of Condolence from His Holiness Daniel, Patriarch of Romania, *Read at the Funeral Service of Mioara Grigore* 232

CONTENTS

Appendix 1: "Sacrificing Oneself for Another Is an Overwhelming Miracle" *Interviews with Mioara and Viorel in 2013*. 235

Appendix 2: "I Would Die from the Happiness of Being Able to Live!" *An Interview with Mioara and Viorel in 2014*. . 252

Appendix 3: "I'm Not Alone—I'm with Mioara" *Interviews with Viorel and Maria in 2016* 266

Editor's Preface

In March of 2016, we received a query from a Romanian pilgrim to our monastery in California, asking if we would be interested in publishing a book translated from Romanian. As we learned from our pilgrim, this book with a paradoxical title, *Cancer, My Love,* had become greatly loved throughout Romania since its publication there in March 2014. The book was the memoir of a mother of five, Mioara Grigore, who had struggled with cancer.

We contacted the book's editor, Anca Stanciu, who was also one of the editors of the magazine *Familia Ortodoxă* (The Orthodox Family) and a close friend of Mioara at the end of her life. She told us something that helped explain the book's popularity: "As I wrote in the foreword,[1] Mioara was like a magnet, a magnet of love—and now I understand this was her gift from God. Everybody felt so happy by her side. And this love radiates from the book."

But there was another reason for the book's impact: its transformative power. Mioara was a person who felt things intensely and deeply. A priest who knew her has said, "I believe God gave Mioara an extraordinary affective

---

[1] See p. 14 below.

[emotional] memory."[2] Happily, she was also possessed of a remarkable ability to capture in words the feelings she remembered, to convey them vividly to the reader. And she had a story to tell, a story of personal transformation. Although Mioara would never have called herself a "magnet of love," it's clear from the testimony of those who knew her that she *became* such precisely through such experiences as were related in this book. In her account, she was quite candid about her weaknesses and fears, her temptations and doubts. Nevertheless, she described how, with help from God and her loved ones, she was able not only to persevere, but also to learn and grow spiritually by means of her greatest challenges. Her retelling of events was so striking, and at the same time so authentic, that the reader could feel along with her, and moreover *learn* along with her. In this way, the lives of countless people have been changed. As Anca wrote to us, "In Romania we've seen miracles with this book."

The book is a testament to the Christian teaching that sickness, which entered the world together with death as a consequence of sin, is allowed by God for our spiritual purification and perfection. Mioara, although she was a religion teacher by profession, didn't explain this theological point in her book. Her life was the lesson.

A book written by an Orthodox Christian wife and mother, chronicling her struggle with cancer, might have been expected to have a limited appeal, reaching niche markets of

---

[2] See p. 230 below.

believers (especially women with families), cancer patients, etc. In Romania, however, interest quickly spread by word of mouth, and the book was read with profit by people of all backgrounds and circumstances: non-believers as well as believers, married and single, laypeople and monastics, young and old, healthy and sick, those with little education and the highly educated.

A year after the book's publication, Mioara received an award of distinction from the Patriarch of Romania. She lived to witness the book's immense success, and was able to respond to many of those whose hearts were touched by it. As Anca said, however, "She lived all this with humility. She used to say that she was feeling so ill after these times of recognition that she couldn't be proud at all!"

To this English edition of the book, we have added material that was published separately by Anca in *Familia Ortodoxă*. The epilogue is a four-part article that came out shortly after Mioara's repose and that discusses, among other topics, Mioara's final days. Appendix 1 is a two-part interview with Mioara and her husband Viorel conducted in 2013, a year before the book was published. In Appendix 2, the two are interviewed again, this time in May 2014, two months after the book's release. Finally, Appendix 3 consists of interviews with Viorel and with the Grigores' oldest child, Maria, conducted in March 2016, a year after Mioara's repose.

Besides filling in details and providing a continuation of the story, the added material fulfills another important function: it reveals Mioara *as others saw her*. The words of Anca and Viorel after Mioara's repose are especially pertinent in this regard.[3] Here we see the fruit of everything Mioara had learned from her sorrows and joys—and particularly from her sorrows that had turned into joys. It was the fruit not only of what she described in the book but also of what she could not put into words. It was the fruit, too, of what occurred in her soul during her last year, after the book came out, as God continued to purify her, to prepare her for the life beyond. There, in that future life, all the "magnets of love" will find their true home, for there reigns the supreme Source of love, Who draws all unto Himself (cf. John 12:32).

It is our hope and prayer that readers of this English edition of *Cancer, My Love* will reap the benefit of the author's life-story of transformation, for the sake of their own lives, both in this world and in the world to come.

—Abbot Damascene
St. Herman of Alaska Monastery
Platina, California

NOTE: All the footnotes in the main text, epilogue, and appendices are by the editors and translators of the English edition.

---

[3] See the epilogue and Appendix 3.

Foreword
About All Sorts of Gravitational Forces

The hilltop monastery was celebrating its patron saint one spring day. The celebration of the beloved Apostle of Christ filled us all with a different depth, vision, and understanding. The blue and bright sky, the gentle sun, the green meadow ... and in this huge, holy solemnity, our children were running, as if thrown in all directions by an untiring centrifugal force. We were all chasing them feverishly, breathlessly, not knowing who was whose, or whether or not they had fallen into some ravine or had been stuck with a nail, because there were so many building materials around.

Suddenly—I stopped. On the green meadow, in the middle of that race, another image opened in front of my eyes, as if someone had pulled a curtain slightly. Five children with heavenly eyes sat quietly on a blanket. They were not screaming, not struggling, not raging, and—what was even more surprising—they were not even forced not to do so. They looked around, but in their eyes, there was no curiosity, no fidgeting, no unruliness—just a kind of serene and undisturbed wonder, a suspended expectation, an unshakable good. What was keeping them in such peace?

Perhaps another kind of centrifugal force, much stronger than the one spinning our children into a crazy whirlwind.

The same force pulled me toward them, without my being able to resist. In front of them, I found myself telling their mother shyly, "You have wonderful children!"

There, close to them, I began to understand. It was the force of love. The force that drew me certainly flowed from the mother, and it was so powerful that it could surely move the earth from its axis, if need be. I watched them. They were not of this world. From their large eyes, strikingly serene and undisturbed, to their vintage outfits, long silk dresses, fastened with lace and ribbons, wide-brimmed hats covering blond curls, and quiet smiles. They seemed as if from a dream, one of those dreams so exciting, that you do not have the time to realize that you are sleeping.

However, instead of any greeting or "good day," their mother cried, begging, "Pray for me ... I have cancer!"

* * *

That was the day I met Mioara. Like a journey between several strikingly contrasting sceneries that changed instantaneously. From nadir to zenith and then again to nadir. With no shades of gray: with her, you either laughed hard or cried hard. What remained unchanged and stable was the force of attraction that gathered everyone around her, like a magnet—from her husband, to children, friends, and those who read her book now.

FOREWORD

In fact, the entire book can be glimpsed from this meeting of ours. Enchanting scenery, suddenly interchanged with waiting rooms in various hospitals; positive and highly positive characters in a battle against the black and hairy cells of cancer lurking at the corners of lungs and breasts; complicated formulas cunningly describing equations of various gravitational accelerations, from falling into latrines (and all sorts of other toilets) to "falling in love" and in awe as she fell over her husband. Mioara, with her schoolgirl smile, would grasp later that people could fall only where they are placing their center of gravity. "For where your treasure is, there will your heart be also" (Matthew 6:21).

Mioara's path in life, both the real one and the one written here, was a huge effort to move the center of her own existence from her own self, narrow as a dungeon, in which she had been struggling hopelessly, to others first, and then to God. And so, according to all laws of gravitational attraction, both earthly and spiritual, her fallings come to be, finally, the long-awaited fall upwards.

Containing thus a genuine therapeutic method, this book is a medicinal book. Not just a "place to hit your head against" (a place made of someone else's pain), a place that by hitting against you forget all your own sorrows; this book is even more: it is a cure that neutralizes any of your pains from the moment you absorb someone else's pain as yours. Even those of the doctor who, in his inability to do good, does evil—he is the most miserable of all.

That is why, dear reader, you must not leave this book in the library, but put it in your first-aid kit. Toothaches, heartaches, soul aches—everything will be anesthetized once you start to walk on the path followed by the author: prayer for others and not for yourself.

And you can start today: with Mioara.

—Anca Stanciu

ROMANIAN PRONUNCIATION GUIDE

â and î	As the "i" in "sill."
ă	As the "u" in "hurt."
ș	sh
ț	ts

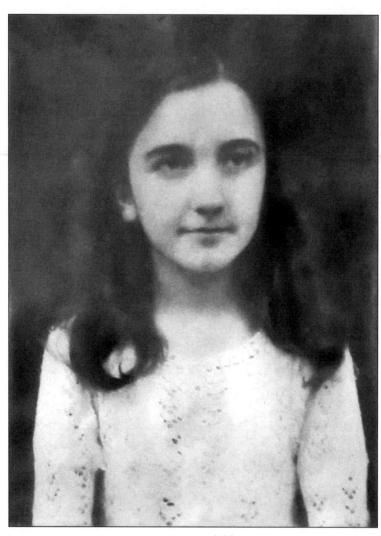

Mioara as a child.

I

The Fall

I CAN still remember. I was falling and falling and couldn't stop, as if life itself was an immense and endless fall.

I was seven years old. I was a very slim, fragile, pale and sensitive little girl.

I remember perfectly. I was playing with some children, slightly older than me, in a deserted backyard, in a village near Târgoviște. It was a hot summer afternoon. God, it was hot! I remember that on that morning my grandmother had braided my hair into pigtails, which I completely detested.

I didn't know then that exactly those pigtails would more or less help to save my life.

I was wearing a white lace dress and I wasn't wearing any shoes. I was barefoot because we were very poor, but it didn't matter.... We loved each other deeply, and, in those days, that love clothed everything in a great richness.

I see these images passing extremely fast in front of my eyes. I was running toward the back of the yard, heading with amazing speed toward an old and deserted latrine. I was running and running with an inexplicable desire to reach that place as soon as possible. It was drawing me like a magnet. Even now, after forty years, my memories are still fresh.

Although I wish they had faded with time, I've never managed to forget.

All those memories hurt, but they have lived with me, have been in me, have breathed through my being, and I have not been able to take them out of my soul.

They still hurt, those moments, but maybe it's for the best like this. To live and relive the nightmare, not being able to forget anything, to relive eternally those feelings.

I finally reached that latrine and I sat hastily on its floor. I still cannot explain how all of a sudden I heard a loud noise, as loud as if the entire world had collapsed under my feet.

The floor below me broke into pieces, and I was falling and falling, an endless fall, trying desperately to clench onto the mud walls until I finally reached the bottom of that immense hole full of excrement and worms.

The impact was so strong that initially I could see only black before my eyes. I remember how I was struggling, I was struggling continuously, and slowly my sight began to clear.

I was surrounded by mud, feces, worms, leaves, cigarette butts, paper, and especially by that fetid smell of human dirt. My little feet were trying to find a support, but there was nothing; I kept moving them with great desperation. My hands were frantically trying to cling to something, but the mud walls of the latrine seemed to continually crumble on me.

I remember that the struggle seemed eternal; a struggle uneven and unjust at the same time. I was struggling with a mountain of refuse and I had no chance to win. I thought I was losing my mind. I had nothing to cling to. I was looking for something to support me, and I could not find anything stable that could truly hold me.

I also remember beginning to run out of air. I had so little air, always insufficient, just like now, when I write this, decades later.

I still have no air, I still do not know how to apportion it well, but my memories are sufficient, painful enough.

I continued to struggle. That huge and stinking sea of sewage started to cover me completely. Occasionally I pushed down that viscous and smelly filth with my legs and managed to briefly lift my head above the surface. The sewage had covered me completely. It had entered my mouth, nose, ears, eyes. I was full of it everywhere.

I could not breathe, I could not scream for help, no matter how much I wanted to. I was getting tired. I was drowning. I was drowning within that giant fetid mass of dirt and I could not breathe, I could not cry for help. The ordeal was beyond imagination. I had no strength to move my hands or feet. My mouth was full of human waste, my whole being was full of waste, and then I started to float. I just wanted to sleep, to rest. I was slowly giving up. I stopped struggling. I stopped fighting and I let myself go down to the bottom of the pit, where death was waiting for me with its awful smell of excrement. I closed my eyes as I was letting myself be swallowed by that pit full of worms, when miraculously something scratched my cheek. It scratched me so hard that it made me open my eyes. A tree branch came out of nowhere. With a last effort, I stretched out my hands and managed to cling to that branch.

As I did so, I released a blood-curdling scream, the scream

of an animal escaping from slaughter, a scream that forced enough waste matter out of my mouth to allow for some air in. My scalp started to ache. Someone was pulling me up by my pigtails. Back to light, back to air, back to life. I did not let go of the branch. (For days I slept with that branch next to me, the branch that brought me back among the living.)

I was finally taken out. People gathered around me, as if they had seen a ghost.

A hose with a spray of cold water was used to quickly wash me. (I have loved water so much ever since!) And that was the day when my "cruddy"[1] life came to an end.

The fact is that my struggle in that latrine, when I was seven, was my redeeming torment, my piece of eternity, God's miracle in my life when I least expected it. I always used to think that my struggle with death in that latrine was the most serious and difficult moment of my life.

Hardly has it been so.

In my life, I have understood one thing: that branch that saved me when I was seven, turned up, in one form or another, at the most terrible moments of my life. All I had to do was to recognize it as a miracle.

But many years had to pass before I came to understand this, and moreover a lot of pain had to pass—a lot of pain.

---

[1] Here the author uses a word that denotes something insignificant or trivial, i.e., that could be thrown into the garbage or latrine.

2

Stairs

Years passed.... What had I been doing all this time?

Schools, college, university ... all kinds of books that I shouldn't have read, all sorts of moments that I shouldn't have lived ... chunks of time irreversibly lost.

I had been living in an unreal world. I had had an unnaturally prolonged childhood. I could not part with my parents, no matter how old I was. I used to fall in love all the time with characters from books or movies, and I used to imagine what it would have been like if I had lived dozens or even hundreds of years ago.

I was a hopeless dreamer, and what hurt me most was that I could not grow up at all. I was stuck somewhere in a time loop and I could not escape from it.

Time was running implacably and I was anchored somewhere outside it.

At thirty I was still the same foolish girl, with my dreams, with my books, still in my own world.

I was thirty when I had my first encounter with heartbreaking pain, that overwhelming pain caused by the loss of someone loved. My father was dying. I adored him. He was everything to me. I had an amazingly beautiful and gentle father, a man of rare dignity. He would rather suffer for months, or even years, than offend or humiliate someone.

He had a rare spirit of sacrifice. I would have moved mountains not to lose him.

In the mornings I was going to Pitești to work, in the afternoons I was going to classes at the University in Târgoviște, and at nights I was catching whichever train I could to Bucharest, just to see him at the Fundeni hospital, if only for a few moments.

He had cirrhosis. I was crying all the time. When I was hitchhiking, when I was waiting for the train, when I was waiting for the subway. I was crying everywhere. Crying and begging God to let me have him for a little longer.

One winter night, I helped him sit up and I hugged him as if he were a small child.

"I feel like throwing up," my father said to me, looking me in the eyes with unimaginable love. A little later, he vomited blood and tissue into my hands. The next day he died. And with him, a part of me died as well.

In my father, I saw the best of humanity, that innocent, pure, sincere, angelic part.

He never scolded me, never slapped me. He only gave me love, love, and love.

I always wondered how it was possible for a human being to be so patient, so gentle. And, what hurt me most was that, unfortunately, I didn't even remotely resemble him. I wanted so badly to have some of his gentleness.

His disappearance shook me so much that I decided to go for a Confession for the first time in thirty years.

STAIRS

Through a combination of more than favorable circumstances, on a torrid summer day, I found myself before Fr. Arsenie Papacioc.[1]

His cell was redolent with holiness, and Father's gentle and angelic presence gave me the courage to confess my sins.

When I told him my age and that I was not married, Father asked me, a little surprised, "What if you had a car accident and died? What would you have left behind?" I did not respond. It made me think.

I had never thought about my own death. I thought years were mine and I had all the time in the world. After an hour, I went out, astonished and overwhelmed, as if a new heart were beating in my chest. I felt I was someone new.

A cool summer rain had started and I stretched out my hands, as if wishing for my whole being to be washed. The Holy Confession had washed away my sins; that summer rain was washing my body.

O God! If only I could have kept myself as I was on that summer day! What if I could have known then what was to come in my life?

I was thirty-four when, on a beautiful autumn day, I fell down some stairs, stairs that would change my life irrevocably

---

[1] Archimandrite Arsenie Papacioc was one of the holy elders of modern-day Romania who, having been tried by suffering in the Communist prisons, shone with Christ-like love and compassion. Over the course of several decades, multitudes came to him for spiritual counsel. He reposed on July 17, 2011, at the age of ninety-seven, at the Dormition Convent in Techirghiol (southeast Romania), where he had served as spiritual father. Over ten thousand people were present at his funeral.

CANCER, MY LOVE

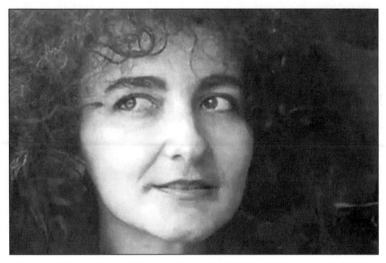

Mioara as a young woman.

and completely. It was September 15, my first day as a newly appointed teacher at a high school in Tărtășești. It was the first day of the school year. I was wearing a long blue dress. I had an abundance of curly hair and green eyes, and I weighed forty-five kilos.[2] My soul was full of hopes and dreams. I was still a dreamer, a foolish, clumsy girl, and above all a misfit.

For some reason, that day I received more flowers than I had ever received in my life. The students welcomed me with questions and smiles, and our vivid discussions lasted for a long time. At the end of the school day, I was on the first floor, with dozens of flowers in my arms and a pair of high heels on my feet, when I managed to get tangled in my own skirt and to fall ... and fall.... And, O God! I felt that I landed on

[2] About ninety-nine pounds.

someone. My dress was long and large. That person was under my dress, I was over him, the flowers were on top of us both, and my heart was racing, ready to burst out of my chest.

I blushed. A redheaded, well-built man appeared from under my dress, and I recognized him as the mathematics teacher. I asked him, almost panting with embarrassment, "Are you hurt, Professor? I'm Mioara. You know, I'm the new teacher, and I have a name you'd give to a sheep," I said with a slight smile.[3]

"Viorel," he said, offering me a strong hand, "and I have a name you'd give to an ox."[4]

We both laughed heartily. He helped me get up, we collected the flowers from the floor, and that was how my first day as a teacher ended.

All the way home on the bus, I was accompanied by a terrible shame, the shame of making a fool of myself. That night I was tense and upset with myself.

I was hoping to be perceived by my peers as being sober, strong, dignified, and full of mystery.

Instead I had left the impression that I was a loser. How many times did I have to fall in this life of mine?

I woke up in the morning and decided to put it behind me and start fresh. I was already missing my students. The first teacher I met in the teachers' lounge was the math teacher. He had a chess set under his arm. His presence embarrassed me

---

[3] In Romanian, "Mioara" is a name, but also a noun that can mean "sheep."

[4] "Viorel" is a name that Romanians commonly give to their male children, but also that peasants frequently given to their oxen.

and annoyed me at the same time. Firstly, because I couldn't stand redheaded men and, secondly, because he was reminding me of how I had fallen over him. But there was nothing I could do. A new journey was about to begin that day, a journey that led me up and down at the same time. That day I was about to begin my famous ...

3

Sicilian Defense[1]

I WALKED IN with a forced smile. When he saw me, he said that he would really like to play a game of chess with me. At that time, I did not know how obsessed he was with this game. Unfortunately, I was too. I had spent years, in my childhood, waiting for my father to come back from work so we could play chess till the early hours.

I had spent most of my youth caught in the spell of this game.

The feeling of winning a game was truly something. I felt as if on a battlefield, a soldier and a general at the same time.

After school hours, we started to play. I had a huge desire to win and to humiliate him in public. I succeeded with the first game. The other teachers laughed at him. I rejoiced. After a few games, he started to play for real. He started to beat me with humiliating scores and he proposed to play for money. We looked at each other like two criminals and I accepted. He beat me completely. I had to give him my bus money. That day I walked five kilometers to get home. I swore that I would

---

[1] In chess, the Sicilian Defense is the most popular and best-scoring response to White's first move. It was first recorded by two Italian chess players in the sixteenth century.

seek vengeance. My feet were swollen and hurt awfully. From that day on, I started to make chess the purpose of my life. I lived only to win. At night, I was studying Fischer and Kasparov. After a few days, I started to win. Each game was a great challenge for me. The other teachers were circling us. Slowly, I started to win. I was winning the chess games, but I was blind to the fact that he was actually winning something else: territory in my heart, and time—precious time. He had a brilliant plan to conquer me, for he was a good mathematician. He had indestructible logic, and I was just naive—naive with a capital N.

One day I asked the school principal if he knew anyone who was lodging people. The commute was terribly tiresome. Immediately, he told me of a teacher who had a big old house, like a mansion, for lease. He said, "Let me show him to you, he's in the teachers' lounge." He pointed him out to me and I froze. It was my chess opponent. This situation annoyed me no end, because by then I resented him. But there was no way to pull out, so we agreed to go and see the place.

It was a rainy autumn day. He led me to an old gate, and invited me in. I was so angry that I kicked the gate wide open with my knee. He would later tell me that it was exactly that kick in the gate that made him fall in love with me. "You were some woman … my whole life I had been looking for such a woman!"

I didn't know what he meant at the time.

The rain was getting heavier. We could not go inside the house because the teacher said he had forgotten the keys, so he ceremoniously invited me into the barn. At the back of the garden, he had a big barn with a long ladder leaning into it. It was raining cats and dogs, and I was soaked to my skin. So I climbed the ladder into the famous edifice. While climbing, I remembered St. John Climacus' *Ladder of Divine Ascent* and asked the teacher if he had read it. Wet and puzzled, he replied that at the age of thirty-five he had read only Emil Cioran.[2]

I was more than disappointed. "What an uncultivated teacher," I said to myself. "What am I doing in his barn?" Inside, the hay gave me a feeling of warmth and comfort. I sat on a stack of hay. So did the redheaded teacher. I was extremely anxious, so I started talking quickly about the Egyptian *Paterikon*,[3] especially about St. Anthony the Great and about his ascetic struggles.

He suddenly interrupted me and told me bluntly, "I'm crazy about you. I think I'm in love with you."

I looked at him confused. His remark offended me and I found it humiliating that he was not paying any attention to what I was saying. All I wanted was to go down the ladder immediately. The air in the barn was suddenly suffocating. I realized we were from completely different worlds.

I set foot on the first step of the ladder, and the redheaded teacher came after me with a desperate air and tried to hug me. A rainbow of surreal beauty appeared just then in the sky, coloring it in thousands of shades.

---

[2] A Romanian existentialist philosopher and essayist, who published works in Romanian and French (1911–1995).

[3] A *Paterikon* is a collection of biographies and teachings of saints, arranged according to a particular country, region, or monastery.

I hit him so hard that I almost fell, along with the ladder, from a considerable height.

"I would never hurt you—don't you understand?" I could hear him saying before I got down quickly and ran away. I ran and ran, I didn't know where to. In fact, I don't think I was running away from him, but from myself. But I was too proud to admit it then. "I know by heart the life of St. Anthony the Great ... he knows nothing," I said to myself. "He's superficial and uncultivated," I consoled myself. "How could I waste my time with him?"

When I arrived home, I wanted to fall asleep as quickly as possible, but I couldn't. I was so agitated, and my broken dreams that night were all about haystacks, barns, and especially ladders—ladders that went nowhere.... I was climbing them and wasn't getting anywhere. In my dreams I was oppressed by a terrible sadness. And I still remember that I was climbing alone on those ladders.

God, how alone I was!

4

The Pilgrimage

THE DAYS passing by were all the same. Or, at least that's what I wanted to believe. At school, I was trying to carry on as unnoticed as possible. I wasn't speaking at all with the redheaded teacher, until one day when he asked me briefly what he could do so that I would stop being mad at him. I replied sharply that I would be very happy if he would stop talking to me. He looked at me with so much sadness. I could not stand his look. I had never in my life met such eyes, so tearful, meek and innocent.

"Ox eyes," I said to myself. "His name could have been none other than Viorel! How can a man without faith in God have such an innocent look?" I asked myself, fuming with anger. How could I, such a complex, sophisticated, and mysterious being, with such a complicated and laborious mind, be moved by someone so simple? I became tense again. I was rejecting any thought or feeling about him. I anchored myself again to the thought of St. Anthony the Great. "I'll become a nun one day," I thought, increasingly satisfied with this idea. I was picturing myself somewhere in the mountains, in a shabby cell, lit only by candlelight, praying and making prostrations, while fighting against my own passions, just like my dear saint.

At school, I spent all my breaks with my students. I avoided the teachers' lounge. It was like a minefield to me, and therefore extremely dangerous. Until one day, when I had to grab a grade book, and I saw the teacher smoking anxiously in a corner. Our colleagues, including the principal, were seated around a long table in the middle of the room. When the teacher saw me coming in, he jumped up and, with the cigarette still in the corner of his mouth, he came to me trembling and saying loudly, "I love you madly, what don't you understand?" He was in front of me, looking at me very determined. And then, between the cigarette smoke coming out of his mouth and the smoke coming out of my angry brain, I slapped him in the face, making the cigarette fly to the other end of the table, until it landed right in front of the principal.

There was a deafening silence in the room—everybody froze. The red marks of my fingers could be seen etched on his right cheek like an eternal testimony. He became entirely red. I was almost blowing smoke through my nostrils. I was expecting him to fight back. He was a man, wasn't he?

But it didn't happen. On the contrary, he made a very candid gesture; he covered his cheek with his hand where I had hit him and told me, almost whispering, "Forgive me," before he rushed out.

I remained there in a state of bemusement that to this day I cannot explain.

I felt so ashamed. I had never hit anyone before. I went outside just as quickly as he had, and locked myself in the restroom, where I cried, sitting on the toilet seat. I cried and I cried, thinking that, since I was seven, I had found my agony, tranquility, and release in all sorts of toilets, more or less welcoming and clean.

"A cruddy life," I finally concluded, after releasing all my tears and pressure in that toilet stall. I went out and I started to walk, and I walked and walked, crossing two villages, without stopping for a moment's rest. Who was I running from? I did not know. One thing was certain: if night had not come and I had not gotten scared, I could have kept walking. Looking back now, I realize that I was walking and running so much because I was afraid. I was afraid to be alone with myself, to remain quietly alone with my thoughts.

That night I slept like a rock.

I wanted to sleep for at least a thousand years.

I felt so helpless—a feeling which I disliked deeply, but which grew stronger in my heart.

The following days I took leave from school. On the third day, someone called me at my gate. I looked out the window and could not believe it. It was the redheaded teacher. For the first time, I felt an undefined emotion and a slight shiver of joy when I saw him. "What if I were to apologize to him?" I said to myself, slightly confused by what would happen. I ran to the gate. At the bottom of the stairs I stumbled again (of course) and I fell. Falling was almost part of my nature. I stood up quickly, mechanically arranging some strands of curly hair, and asked him what he wanted. He said that, first of all, I had to return to school the following week, and, secondly, that he had heard I wanted to go on a pilgrimage to St.

Parasceva's holy relics. "Would you like to go with me? I can get hold of a car and we can leave tomorrow."

"With you?" I asked, puzzled. "What do you want to do at the saint's relics? You know nothing about her, you don't believe, you haven't gone to Confession in your life, you don't take Holy Communion.... How do you think you could ..."

He suddenly stopped me, looking at me decisively, and said only four words: "I want to learn."

Again those innocent eyes, which suddenly changed my mood and made me feel, for a moment, an immense compassion. I would have cried for him until exhaustion, until dissolution.

"All right then, tomorrow at 4 p.m. Be here with the car."

I turned around and left him at the gate. Inside me, I hoped that he would not come, that he would not keep his word, proving that he was not capable of anything. I would then congratulate myself that I had won, that he had been nothing but a temptation in the way of my monastic life, and that I had been a thousand times smarter than he, and obviously I would eventually become a nun living in the mountains, facing the vicissitudes of weather and fighting with temptations like St. Anthony, the saint of my youth. But none of that was to happen. The next day, at 4 p.m. sharp, not one minute before or after, he was at my gate, as he had promised. We were both to go on a pilgrimage.

"Lord, don't leave me.... I'm going to a holy place, with an unbeliever. Have mercy, Lord!"

I watched him driving. He was confident. We both kept quiet the whole way. I believe we were so scared of each other that only silence could provide a feeling of safety. We were passing unknown roads, hills, and forests. "Now he could kill me," I thought, imagining all kinds of tenebrous scenarios. A paralyzing fear had frozen me. "One could expect anything from a man who hasn't been for a Confession in his life," I said to myself as beads of sweat began to cover my forehead.

"And what if he cuts me into pieces?" I thought, my mind sunk in despair.

Eventually, tired of being so afraid, I fell asleep. I had a surprisingly reassuring sleep, like I hadn't had for a long time. When I woke up, I could not believe my eyes…. I was in the middle of a city full of lights and nice people. Iași revealed itself to me in its charming beauty. Even the air seemed full of holiness.

We got in line. There were thousands of people waiting.[1] The teacher stood next to me. His shoulder was touching mine. For the first time I had a feeling of safety. I did not feel alone anymore. I looked at him, as he was waiting in line, determined to beat fatigue, doubts, and the multitude of questions I could see in his eyes. He continued to be silent and I was glad that, for the first time, I wasn't alone there, waiting to venerate the saint. Even next to an unbeliever, waiting in line became a true initiation, not only for him, but for me as well.

---

[1] St. Parasceva, an ascetic of the eleventh century, is a beloved saint in the Orthodox countries of Eastern Europe. Hundreds of thousands of pilgrims come every year to her holy relics, treasured in the Metropolitan Cathedral in Iași, Romania, to ask for her heavenly intercessions.

I was given a real life lesson. All my theological pride was shattered by his docility.

"I want to learn." His words still rang in my ears, as a refrain uttered endlessly. "Learn what?" I thought, as if trying to calm myself. "He doesn't understand anything of all this."

But he continued to wait in line, to wait with me with a stubbornness that disarmed me completely, one, two, three, ten, twenty hours until the unavoidable happened....

5
The Fainting Spell

WITH ONLY two hours left before reaching the saint's holy relics, naturally, I fainted. I had been in line for almost twenty hours, tired, hungry, and especially dehydrated, refusing to drink water and eat (of course, because of my pride), so I fainted.

The teacher lifted me in his arms and tried to get me out of the line. There was no way out—we were flanked on both sides by a mass of people. With incredible strength, he took me in his arms and pushed to get me out of there to some fresh air.

As I was feeling better, he reassured me that the following day he would wait in line for me while I slept in the car. But the next day, fresh and determined, we both started queuing all over again.

After endless hours of waiting, when we were only about half an hour from reaching the front, I felt as if I were about to faint again.

"Don't you dare faint again!" he told me, more determined than ever. "You will hold on even if I have to carry you in my arms to the saint!" And he grabbed me by my waist with "atomic" force and held me in his arms and supported me, until I got in front of the saint.

What should I tell her first? What should I ask her for? I thanked her that she made me worthy to come before her, and then I begged her to help me "get rid" of the teacher: "I beseech you, make him disappear from my life, I beg you!"

Mixed feelings and undefined emotions overcame me as I walked away, waiting for the teacher to come out, too.

It seemed like forever until he finally appeared. I could not believe it. His cheeks were flooded with tears, but his face was covered in light. He was beaming with happiness.

"What do you feel?" I asked curiously.

"I don't know the feeling, but it's great!" he said to me, so surprised himself, like one who had just found the secret of immortality a moment ago.

We walked side by side along the streets full of the lights and people of the city.

We didn't say much, but quietly enjoyed the unreal inner joy, and the holiness of those moments.

6

The Spiritual Father

As time passed, I felt more and more caught up with him. Thoughts seemed like they were not my own anymore, but revolved only around his person. I panicked. I ran to my spiritual father and told him that I was struggling with a great temptation. I felt like giving up teaching in that high school. I saw him every day and it made me sick. I felt I had completely betrayed St. Anthony the Great. I felt like a coward. I wanted and at the same time I didn't want to see the redheaded teacher. This struggle was so sweet and challenging!

One day, he invited me to go to Bucharest. "It's a surprise," he told me. I was very curious to see where he would take me.

We arrived in front of Antim Monastery.[1] To my shame, I hadn't been there for many years.

There were many people waiting in front of a monastic cell. We got in line. Fr. Adrian Fageteanu[2] was hearing Confessions and giving blessings for hours. Our turn came after four hours of waiting. The redheaded teacher, who, in only

---

[1] A monastery in Bucharest, built in the years 1713–1715.
[2] Hieromonk Adrian was a Romanian elder who endured many years (1945–1946, 1952–1964) in Communist prisons for his faith. He reposed on September 27, 2011, at the age of ninety-eight.

three months, had turned my entire inner being upside down, went in first. I waited for him to come out, thinking that he wouldn't be in there for long. "What could an engineer talk about with a priest-monk of such spiritual depth?"

One hour, two hours, three hours passed. Worried and intrigued at the same time, I kept marveling at how much humility Father had if he could "waste" so much of his time with an engineer, who had no knowledge about God.

Finally, the teacher came out, brighter and more hopeful than ever. I went in too. I told Father roughly my story.

"I'm teaching religious education at a high school," I said, not without a certain pride in my voice.

"Tell me," he asked with a heavenly gentleness in his voice, "what do you have against this man? Why are you judging him so much?"

"Father," I replied abruptly, "first of all, he's an engineer and he's way too rational, since at the age of thirty-five he doesn't know God, and, secondly, he keeps proposing to me with diabolical insistence. You know, I was thinking of becoming a nun...."

Father looked at me with kindness. The sun had set long ago. Night had fallen slowly over the cells and the light in his eyes seemed to illumine everything around.

"I think you should accept him—he's a man with a very good soul!"

I could not believe it. What could Father have seen in him that I didn't see or refused to see?

"Let's pray for the gift of childbearing. You shall give him five children!"

I thought, Father must be joking.... How is it possible to have five children? I'm already thirty-four....

Prayers followed. They seemed endless. I heard a dozen times: "Viorel and Mioara, Viorel and Mioara...."

The night grew deeper. The stars shone more intensely, silent witnesses to the holiness in that little cell.

Back then, I had no idea what was about to come in my life. I had no idea what a special priest there was in front of me, and I certainly had no idea how his prayers would impact my life. I was speechless, but I felt an inner shiver of anticipation, of an intensity that almost frightened me.

I did not want to accept that feeling, to acknowledge it, to define it, but it had already happened, it was already in me. I had fallen in love. I was about to start a new life. So late, though. It was as if I had been born and had died at the same time. Later that night, we both left Father's cell, dizzy, as if drunk. Drunk with love. I did not think that was possible. I did not think this miracle could be possible for me.

So early, and yet so late....

7

The Wedding

"You'll be my wife, and moreover, we'll have many children," the redheaded teacher told me one day, determined as always. I, naturally, remained speechless. I had to see my spiritual father as quickly as possible.

"Father, he tells me that I'll be almost constantly pregnant, and I can't get rid of him! He wants to marry me at any cost!" And I started to tell him in detail about my struggle (which was almost no longer a struggle) with the great temptation called "the redheaded teacher."

"So, you really love him?" Father asked me quite naturally. After a few moments of silence, I uttered the most determined "YES" in my life. And then, I shouted again, from the deepest corner of my being, "YES!"

I was so ashamed that I had said it, but it also felt so good. I felt relieved.

Outside, it was raining slowly, as if it were never going to stop. Nature itself seemed to call for patience, for infinite patience. But I had no patience. Neither with time, nor with my body, not to mention my soul. I was distraught, overwhelmed, scattered into thousands of pieces, but happy. Happy and joyful. A joy I had never tasted until then. Over the following months, my mind was immersed in hundreds of questions as to whether the joy I felt was "the real thing." Finally, after months of soul-searching and inner struggle, of spiritual turmoil and agony, we went to receive a blessing to get married.

Remorse was accompanying me permanently, remorse in its entire splendor.

"What if I have upset St. Anthony the Great?" I wondered all the time.

I had betrayed him.... What had become of my dream to find refuge in the mountains, to become a nun, to have prayer as my only company? I was not consistent, and this was one of my main shortcomings. I was unstable and vulnerable at the same time. Sometimes I felt an undefined longing, almost unearthly, for St. Anthony's path. And, in those moments, I used to run to my spiritual father and tell him, "I miss him so much."

"If you missed him so much, you wouldn't still be in the world!" Father's reassuring answer always came. Of course, he was right.

And I would return to my world, to my redheaded teacher with gentle eyes—so gentle that I was completely disarmed.

For me he quit smoking, went for Confession, received Holy Communion, and attended the Holy Liturgy on Sundays. And, above all, my spiritual father was surrounding him with so much love. Sometimes I was so jealous. He let himself be humiliated by me so many times, and yet he did not consider it at all humiliating. He was so docile. So I came up with a plan, the final test, I thought.

I remember that day. Winter had begun. It was snowing so

beautifully. Christmas was not far off. Snowflakes were falling over us. We were both white.

"If you truly want me to be your wife, you must agree to adopt a child!" I thought he would not agree to that. "He'll give up the whole thing now," I said to myself. "Then I'll be free to follow my dream. I'll go to the mountains; I'll be with my dear saint again; and, above all, I won't feel that terrible feeling of shame and betrayal."

I felt so free.

I eagerly waited for his answer. I watched him. He had the same kind eyes.

"I'm going to see Father now, but this time by myself!" He left me there, alone in the snow, and departed. He was strong and determined as always.

He came back late in the evening, happier than ever.

"If, after the wedding, you don't get pregnant within one month, then we'll adopt, not one, but ten children!"

Once again, he left me speechless. "I hadn't thought of that! O Lord, my plans crumbled again!" I was and I wasn't happy at the same time.

"Just get married!" Father told us bluntly one day.

And so our wedding date was decided on the spot, for the feast day of St. Maximus the Confessor, on January 21.

It was a small wedding, with a pair of wonderful godparents and a few other guests.[1] I couldn't stop trembling with emotion. It was a beautiful and frosty winter day. I remember

---

[1] In Romanian Orthodox tradition, the bride and groom must choose godparents (nași): an Orthodox couple who will serve as mentors to the newlyweds.

I was wearing only my wedding dress in the church, but it seemed so warm. I kept looking down the whole time. I could not look at the icon of St. Anthony the Great. When I finally looked up, I was startled. It seemed to me that he was looking straight at me with so much love, as I was marrying my redheaded teacher.

Was it good, was it bad? I did not know. I was almost thirty-five years old, and only now was my life actually beginning. But what a life.... Not one life, but a hundred lives, a thousand lives that were exploding in my soul. I was overwhelmed by a multitude of feelings, by the miracle of love that I had the privilege and honor to be a part of.

If only I had known how to fully relish all this evidence of love, but I did not. I was too afraid.

I felt as if I needed to ask for forgiveness that I had dared to fall in love at thirty-four as if I were fourteen. I still felt like a foolish child.

8

The Wedding Night

INEVITABLY, the wedding night came. The image of the two of us on our wedding night is archaic and archetypal at the same time.

I was sitting on the bed, still in my wedding dress, rubbing my hands and crying. My husband was down at my feet, holding my hands in his and asking me candidly and endearingly, "Why are you crying, my love? Are you afraid?"

"No, I'm not afraid," I answered between two hiccups. "It's just that I desperately miss …"

"Whom do you miss, my love?" asked my adorable and puzzled husband.

"My mother!" I answered, almost drowning in tears.

She was somewhere in a village about seventy kilometers away. She had been too sick to come to our wedding. Her absence hurt me immensely. My unnaturally prolonged childhood had invaded my wedding night as well.

I could not sleep without my mother. That was my great tragedy. For thirty-four years I had slept in the same bed with my mother. The rest was only silence, as my friend Hamlet said.

As I was sitting on the bed, crying over the absence of my mother, my husband did something that stunned me. At three o'clock in the morning he went to a neighbor, woke him up, and begged him to lend us his car.

And so, on our wedding night we ventured, through a numbing frost, on a most fascinating journey. The journey toward a mother's grieving heart. Toward an old and sick woman who was not able to see her only daughter get married.

It was snowing so thickly that we could not see more than one meter in front of us. My huge white wedding dress filled a quarter of the car and covered half of my husband. I tried to temper my heartbeats, and I shuddered at the thought of my mother's warm and maternal embrace, of her eyes, so blue and so amazed when, at 4 a.m., she would see at the door her daughter in her wedding dress.

But, in the whitest night I had ever seen, while it was snowing so impetuously, in a village about halfway there we ran out of gas.

We had a "no gifts" wedding, so all we had with us were a few pennies.[1] Still, to our great joy, we could see the flashy sign of a gas station about one kilometer further down the road. We got out of the car extremely determined, and we both began to push it towards the gas station.

Suddenly, from out of nowhere, men and women appeared in the street, started to point at us, and laughed and shouted to one another, "Look there, look how the bride pushes the car!"

Somewhat proud of myself, I pushed harder. I had no idea that I had such strength.

---

[1] Traditionally, in Romania the newly married couple receives money from the guests at their wedding.

Finally, we refueled and managed to arrive at our destination. I began to shout at the gate, "Mom, Mom, Mommy, open. It's me, Mioara, your daughter!"

No answer. Nothing but silence, wind, and the drifting snowstorm.

We began to strike the gate strongly.

Finally, a light was switched on inside the house, and my mother came out onto the porch, shouting into the cold night with great worry in her voice, "Is it you, my doll?"

"Yes, mother, it's me …"

My mother hadn't seen Viorel yet. He was somewhere behind the car. So, with the same worry in her voice, she shouted back, loud enough for half the village to hear, "What is it, my child? Did he not find you in the proper way? Did he send you away?"

In this expression, "in the proper way," I instantly recognized the entire ancient tradition of the Romanian people.[2]

"No, Mom, we simply wanted to see you tonight," I reassured my mother, whose face suddenly brightened with relief and happiness as she invited us inside.

We brought some cozonac[3] and some sarmale[4] from the

---

[2] In Romania, particularly in the countryside, "Did he not find you in the proper way?" would be an idiomatic way of asking a bride if she had been found to be not a virgin on her wedding night. In the villages, especially in the past, the husband could send the bride away in such a case.

[3] A traditional Romanian and Bulgarian sweet leavened bread, which is a type of stollen.

[4] Stuffed cabbage rolls, usually made with minced meat and rice.

car, and all three of us sat at a small table, in the little shabby house where I had spent almost thirty-five years.

It was the happiest night of my life. I was with the two people I loved the most, and I was about to begin the story of my life, a life that would outlive its time.

I was no longer thirty-five years old. I had a completely different age. The age of a great love.

9

The Birth of the First Child— Gray-Eyed Maria

I HAD NOT believed him. How could I have believed him? My husband told me almost prophetically, "You'll be pregnant within a month!"

Less than a month after our wedding, at the venerable age of thirty-five, I told him, not without a certain tremor in my voice, that we would have a baby. The news fell like a thunderbolt. He took me in his arms and spun me in a mad rush. He started to spoil me like a princess. He almost annoyed me by asking the same question all the time: "My love, what do you want to eat? Is there anything you're craving for?"

What more could I crave for? I already had everything. I had so much love! And on top of that, we had a special place of our own. My husband had inherited from his grandparents a hundred-year-old house, an old-style building, with window shutters. It became our home, a home where time stopped being linear. It felt as if we were somewhere in eighteenth-century Russia.

Every day when my husband left for school, as he locked

the heavy iron gate, I felt like a secluded princess, waiting for her knight. I loved this game.

All my life I had longed for a knight on a white horse to take me to his castle. I already had the knight, even if he had no horse, but a Trabant,[1] and for his kingdom, a small piece of land, where we planted some potatoes. But those iron gates made me feel like some special princess.

It had been almost three months since our wedding, and my belly began to grow. Then, on a warm spring afternoon, I woke up with a full and unstoppable bleeding.

We were so frightened by the prospect of losing our child that I did not even dare to get out of bed.

I didn't want to go to the hospital—I was scared to see a doctor. When I started turning blue, my husband took me in his arms and rushed me to a hospital in Bucharest. When we got there it was already night.

I desperately held my belly, begging for the mercy of the Theotokos[2] to spare my child's life. The doctor on duty welcomed me with a warm, reassuring smile. Her smile gave me a little courage for the first time. I looked at her closely. She was blond and beautiful. I started to lose my faith in her. Blond, beautiful, and smart. It seemed too much for just one person.

However, she had a great impact in my life.

She smiled again at me, and examined me with infinite care. The hardest part was when she referred me to have an ultrasound to see if the baby's heart was still beating.

---

[1] A very shabby model of automobile, made in East Germany before the fall of the Berlin Wall.

[2] The Virgin Mary, Mother of God; literally, "God-birthgiver."

I was in a sinister hospital hallway, in a gray hospital shirt, looking terrified, while waiting to hear our baby's heart. And then, then I heard it. It was like heavenly music to my ears. So much happiness! Life sounded so fresh and harmonious! Love produced sounds of unearthly beauty. My husband and I were crying, holding each other and filled with boundless happiness. That sinister hospital hallway now seemed like a little piece of paradise. The rhythmic and lively heartbeats of our child would accompany us for a long time. They gave us so much courage and hope. But I was such a coward, and I was still afraid. I still had no confidence in the infinite goodness of God.

This would be and remain the mistake of my life.

The due date was approaching amazingly fast. Throughout the remainder of the pregnancy, I had by my side the doctor from that night, that beautiful human being, Dr. Raluca.

I could not believe how warm and full of sacrifice she was. A true fighter, she was almost the only one in that hospital who refused to perform abortions.

"I will never cut little hands and feet," she said, "even if they fire me." In the end, she did have to leave that hospital, mainly because of me, because she undertook immeasurable risks to save my life at the birth of another child.

Anyway, nine months passed, and one day my contractions started. She told me to come immediately to the hospital. My husband was with me, my teddy bear, as I called him. The contractions grew increasingly in intensity. After about ten hours, during some violent contractions, I strongly clenched him by his shirt and ripped off all the buttons. "Go," I screamed at him, "pray and read the Paraklesis to the Theotokos,[3] because I can't endure it anymore."

It seemed to me that I was the most sinful person in that ward. All the other women were managing to give birth after eight or ten hours—only I was continually screaming, as I could not reach the necessary ten centimeters dilation. I was stuck at around two centimeters, as if my whole being were only breathing through those two centimeters. My soul became so small, about two centimeters small. I could not understand this inhumanly long labor. Ten hours passed, then fifteen, and nothing happened. Suddenly, my husband came back to the delivery room like a tornado and in between my screams told me that he would go to Ghighiu Monastery, to pray at the wonderworking icon of the Theotokos.

I looked at him angrily, with my eyes popping out. At that time, he seemed to me the only one responsible for that long labor. "Go!" I screamed back at him. "And don't return unless you're bringing me a miracle.... I can't endure this much longer."

He looked at me with immense pity. I also felt pity for his pity. With his torn shirt, with bristly hair, unshaven, sleepless and hungry, he looked more pathetic than I did. After almost twenty hours of labor, I started to scream directly to the Mother of God. I think I called for her help tens of times until an outraged nurse came in and completely prohibited me from screaming "theological phrases" like that. "What? Are

---

[3] A supplicatory service to the Mother of God, consisting of a canon, psalms, hymns, and—if a priest is present—ektenias (litanies).

you giving us lessons of faith? You enjoyed making love—now put up with the consequences. You're not the only one giving birth!"

But I could no longer carry on. My physical strength was gone when my doctor went to call the hospital manager. He gave me a very sympathetic look, and, seeing the state I was in, finally agreed to an epidural. While I was receiving the injection in my spine, I managed to thank him and told him through my pain and jerky breaths that he looked a lot like Othello from the Shakespearean play of the same name. He smiled broadly and confessed that nobody had told him that before, especially during labor. "It will be okay," he reassured me, and disappeared as quickly as he had come. I started to scream again. My husband came back exhausted but with a spark of hope in his eyes. Our little miracle was not too far away. After twenty-two hours of labor, the long-awaited baby came out. The doctor gasped, which, in those tense moments, made me think of something very bad and very serious. What could have happened? Had I given birth to such a sick child? Why had the doctor almost screamed?

"She's so beautiful!" she said with a bright smile. "In all these years I've attended countless deliveries, but I've never seen a child with gray eyes.... Such amazing eyes...."

She was holding a small baby girl with curly black hair, weighing three and a half kilos.[4] The doctor gently gave her to me.

I looked at the baby. Indeed, she had gray eyes. She looked

---

[4] About 7.7 pounds.

as if she had come straight from heaven. I held her in my arms. It was as if I were holding paradise and not a baby.

The girl could only be named Maria. A miracle with gray eyes. Daddy became dumb with happiness. "Is this my girl?" he asked, unable to believe his eyes. The baby had been placed by a nurse in a cot, next to my bed. And then, inexplicably, Maria, born a few hours before, turned her head toward her father's voice. She recognized her father by his voice. I was watching that scene of immense love with a peace in my soul that I had not felt for a long time. If only time would stop there.... It was as if eternity were enclosed in those moments. An eternity of love between heaven and earth, an eternity of love between father and daughter.

10

Holy Baptism

THREE DAYS later, we left the hospital with our gray-eyed Maria, with me holding her tightly to my chest. We felt a shiver of anxiety, and, not having the patience to wait for forty days, we decided to baptize her after only eight days. Outside there was a numbing frost! However, the baptism brought us so much tranquility and warmth in our souls, it was as if we had baptized her on a hot summer day. Now, we felt everything was as it should be in our lives. But this state of tranquility would not last for too long.

Around 5 a.m. on the morning of December 7, the feast day of St. Philothea, we went to the Monastery of Curtea de Argeș.[1] It was snowing densely and there was so much snow on the road that, when leaving the house, I told my husband, "I'm scared. The baby is so small. There's so much snow.... If something happens to us …"

"Where is your faith, wife?" he replied, more determined than ever to reach the saint's sepulcher. We got in the car—me

[1] The Holy Martyr Philothea lived at the beginning of the thirteenth century near Veliko Tarnovo in present-day Bulgaria. Her relics are treasured at the Monastery of Curtea de Argeș in south-central Romania, where she is widely venerated as a miracle-working intercessor.

with dark doubts in my soul, and Viorel with the desire to reach our destination. After about an hour of driving, our car predictably stopped. It was an old Oltcit,[2] from which one could not expect too much. As always, I panicked. The heating system of the car stopped, too.

"My love, don't worry, I'll go on foot to look for a gas station and get some help. Stay with the girl in the car and hold her tightly to your chest. Pray to St. Philothea." I watched him disappear into the snow, behind billions of snowflakes.

Inside the car, the cold was slowly creeping in. All I could see through the window was snow. The endless white outside threw me into a terrible state of agitation. I was holding my baby girl really tight, and was blowing hot air into her face and pinching her cheeks and nose all the time. I covered her with my body and continuously implored the mercy of God. I couldn't control my heartbeat. It was as if everything went crazy. I wanted to get out in the snow with the baby and run. I didn't know where to.

I don't remember how long I waited in that state of terrible fear until I heard some taps on the window. My husband was back with help, his face all red and covered with snow. He was panting with cold, unable to speak, and he hugged us both with such love and despair. We were both crying with joy, covering our one-month-old baby with kisses, when all she wanted, poor thing, was to sleep.

Finally, we arrived at the saint's monastery and we thanked her for keeping our baby girl alive during this terrible frost,

---

[2] A brand of car produced in Communist Romania in the 1980s.

and we apologized to Maria because God had given her such foolish parents. But we loved each other so much! When we got back home, we watched our little girl sleep, so pure and peaceful, and we imagined heaven for the first time. It could only look like this: the face of a child who is sleeping so peacefully.

11

Anthony—
The Birth of the Second Child

FORTY DAYS after the birth of our first child, I got pregnant again. History repeated itself. Viorel was again in seventh heaven. He was spoiling me.

During the nine months of pregnancy he kept asking me if I was all right, if I felt any contractions. My belly was growing. Of course, I had Dr. Raluca by my side throughout my second pregnancy. To us, she was like an Edelweiss.[1] So unique and special, so warm and so full of sacrifice.... I remember that during the first labor, she held my hand for hours, to the disappointment of the other doctors, who accused her of being too close to patients. That's how she was with me. I felt so honored and privileged at the same time. I felt I did not deserve her friendship.

The term was close. I called my doctor. Her hair was blonder, her smile was bigger, and her heart was more full of sacrifice than ever. Labor began. We both knew from the

---

[1] A rare flower, which grows in remote mountain regions. A national symbol of Austria, Switzerland, Romania, and Bulgaria, it is associated with the rugged beauty and purity of the Alps and Carpathians.

first child that it would be a long, tiring, and exhausting labor.

But, shockingly, it didn't last as long as the first one. After only ten hours of actual screaming, I felt that the baby was rapidly coming into the world, into a new life. "Another strong contraction. Come on, you're doing okay. Hang on a little longer." I felt as if my eyes were literally popping out of my head, and my mouth was so dry, as if thousands of needles were piercing it. A final scream and that was it.

In the hands of the sweetest doctor in the world was a boy of 3.2 kilos.[2] She put him immediately on my chest. A great peace and tranquility took over me almost instantly. I was floating. But this state would not last for very long. When I saw the little one on my chest, I screamed worse than during labor. Not in terror or pain. It was, in fact, a scream of utter amazement, astonishment, as if I had learned just then how to breathe.

The baby had hair so black and bristly, and eyes so big and black, that it seemed he was not from this world!

But what truly amazed me were his eyelashes. They were so long, as if made of lead. They were so thick, heavy and long that I thought he might never be able to open his eyes. I held him tight to my chest. A little later, when my husband saw him, he too was amazed at those unnaturally long lashes. "Are you sure he's not a girl? Ask the nurses to check again. There is no way he's a boy. He's so sweet and delicate."

But he certainly was a boy. One hour after I gave birth,

---

[2] About seven pounds.

I knew what we should name him. His name could be none other than Anthony. I liked to call him often by his name, as it reminded me of my dear saint.

Both children were growing up. I was breastfeeding both; one was on the pillow next to me, while the other one was at my chest. Sleep was a distant memory. But nothing else mattered, because we were so happy and fulfilled. God gave us so much joy. I did not feel tired or sleepy, nor did I have any other earthly concerns.

Our life was shared between Maria and Anthony, Anthony and Maria, until ... until, forty days later, when, quite predictably, there were another two lines on the pregnancy test. I became increasingly heavy with child. My husband took me in his arms and spun me in a crazy whirlwind. "My love, are you sure?... This is the greatest gift ... But ..."

But I had already started to feel a certain fatigue. I was severely sleep deprived most of my time, so I was in a state of floating.

What I knew for sure was that I had to carry on breastfeeding. No matter what happened, as if my life depended on it. I felt as if breastfeeding my children would keep them safe from all the tragedy of life, from all evil, from all the misfortune that could come to them.

I was pregnant while breastfeeding two small children. There was joy in my soul, but from time to time I felt a shiver of anxiety, fear, and despair that I could not explain. All throughout my pregnancy, I felt like something bad was going to happen with my third child.

"These are the pregnancy hormones," my husband would

calm me down. "Everything will be okay and we'll feel like the richest people in the world. You'll see ... everything will be all right." His words would put my mind to rest.

At night, while trying to fall asleep, I pictured our family with three gorgeous and healthy little children. Until ...

12

About Nektarios

THE CONTRACTIONS became stronger and stronger. I immediately called the doctor, and she told me to get to the hospital immediately and she would meet me there. She had so much patience with me. I didn't know what to give her. In fact, I didn't have anything to give her.[1] My husband and I were barely surviving. We felt so indebted to her. When we arrived at the hospital, she led me straight into the delivery room. Labor started. It was increasingly difficult. I had almost no strength left. The doctor was by my side. She wiped the sweat off my forehead, held my hand, and encouraged me continually.

And she kept smiling. I realized then how much power there was in a smile. I gripped the bed frame. It was night, and the stars began to appear one by one. The same long and tiring labor had started.

I was given injections for dilation, for stimulating the contractions, for easing my pain, but nothing helped me.... After one last effort, and calling on all the saints for help, the third baby came into a new life.

[1] It is very frequent in Romania for patients to give a gift or money to the doctor in gratitude. Unfortunately, this can also leave room for abuse and corruption in the medical system.

I felt so liberated and light. I was waiting for a scream, a cry ... but nothing.

The silence felt threatening. My heart almost leapt from my chest. I was so scared. Cold sweat appeared on my forehead. Then, suddenly, the long awaited scream finally came.

But my relief didn't last long as I heard the doctors whispering between themselves: "Yes, you're right, there's no life line on his palm. See, it's missing! And his eyes are so oblique!"

What "oblique eyes"? What "missing life line"? I was not in a palm-reading parlor, I was in a delivery room!

"What's happening?" I asked in panic.

"Nothing, nothing," the doctors answered. "Calm down, it will be fine."

But I felt everything was far from fine. The tension became almost unbearable.

I was taken to another room to rest. I woke up feeling terrible chills. I felt as if the bed were shaking under me. The room was quite warm. I could not understand why I was trembling so badly. Perhaps my heavy and devastating thoughts caused those chills.

"What oblique eyes?" I kept asking.

My other two children had slightly oblique eyes and they were perfectly healthy. And what about that life line? I never checked their little hands to count the lines. My doctor finally came in. In the late autumn evening light, she looked more beautiful, but also sadder than ever. She took both my hands in hers and brought them to her chest. I started to shiver even more. I was expecting all the weight of a Greek tragedy to fall on me.

"My dear lady, the baby has a problem...."

I was annoyed that after so many years, after being by my side in the most difficult and intimate moments of my life, I still hadn't convinced her to call me simply by my first name, Mioara.

She was always so formal.

"What's wrong with my baby?" I asked between terrible shivers.

"He has Down syndrome.... I'm so sorry."

I looked at her. I did not know what to say. I knew nothing of this condition: what it was, what it meant, and if there was any hope or cure.

"It's not something that can be cured," she said, as if hearing my thoughts. "It's a genetic malformation that causes a very serious degree of disability and reduces the life expectancy to a maximum of thirty-five or forty years. Those affected by Down syndrome have an extra chromosome in each cell, so in a way they're born already somewhat old."

She held me tightly in her arms. Finally, she let go and left. I already missed my baby. The need to see him was unbearable.

"He's not on this floor! The handicapped ones are on the next floor." The last words hurt terribly. I went to the second floor and straight to him. He was such a sweet blond child, with beautiful oblique eyes. I covered him with kisses and involuntarily uncovered his arm. I took his little hand and looked at his palm. Indeed, there were only two lines. Even if his life line was missing, he had given us a new life, a new perspective. The perspective of a life with different landmarks of feeling and thinking. He enriched us. But at the time, I didn't think this way. My husband and I were obtuse, desperate, and crying like two fools. We were constantly looking at his little palm, the same palm that would later caress us and tell us, "I love you ... I love you a lot."

"We should call him Nektarios," I thought. "I'll put this child under St. Nektarios's protection."[2]

We had to remain in the hospital for longer. One day, a nurse came in while I was breastfeeding him and said in a threatening voice, "Do you have any idea what to expect?"

"No, I don't," I replied, and my heart once again began to race.

"Well, he won't speak until he's fifteen or twenty, he'll barely walk at about six, and once he reaches teenage years, he'll only sit there with his tongue out. Children like him have a very long tongue. He'll live a maximum of thirty-five years. But I guess that's a good thing, since he'll be such a burden. If you want, I can arrange for you to get rid of him and abandon him here in the hospital. We'll talk."

And she disappeared out the door. I remained speechless, stunned. I almost could not recover from the shock. Why did I have to listen to all of that? I was so impressionable, so vulnerable. Where was my faith, my love for St. Anthony the Great? It all crumbled in an instant. I needed to get some air, so I went outside. I went to the hospital yard and sat down on a

---

[2] St. Nektarios of Pentapolis and Aegina (1846–1920) is a beloved saint of the modern era, known for his prayerfulness and purity, his humility amidst slander and persecution, his writings, and his many miracles both during his lifetime and after his repose.

large rock under a tree. It was a warm autumn day, with gentle breezes. I looked, resigned, at the trees around me. I envied them for not feeling any pain. I had so much pain in my soul. And as soon as I thought that, I felt as if my soul were slowly disappearing, and in its place there was a void—a huge, endless nothingness that filled me, froze me, calcified me completely. I was so cold that I felt chills again, and I could not think of anything. The void intensified and somehow infiltrated every cell of my body with unstoppable force.

"My Lord, don't leave me!" I screamed a silent cry of pain. I knew that feeling. I was terribly afraid of it. It was despondency. It was worse than any physical pain. I tried to get up from that rock but failed to make any movement. I felt paralyzed.

I was so sad that I could not even cry to release some of that pain. I kept sitting on that huge rock, and all I could see in front of my eyes was the image of a child with Down syndrome, walking with his tongue out, unable to speak, without a family and always depending on someone. That image paralyzed me completely. I felt increasingly cold. On that September afternoon, while I was sitting on that rock, something died in me.

With a final effort, I managed to get up from that rock. I passed by women who were breastfeeding healthy and normal children, children without genetic defects. All sweaty and trembling, I went back to my room to look at my baby, and for the first time I felt a thrill of inner joy.

I could not understand how an angel so sweet could have scared and saddened me so much. I felt a fantastic release.

I took my baby in my arms. He seemed so fragile, and he had such almond-shaped eyes. I cuddled him while holding him, almost desperately, to my chest. Suddenly, tears began to flow over him. Sobbing, I asked for forgiveness from God and from him.

The truth is that we had no idea how to care for a disabled child.

The problem was not, in fact, Nektarios's Down syndrome, but that I had allowed a mountain of sadness and hopelessness into my heart. I never thought that losing hope could bring one down so much. It was devastating. I thought it was the worst thing that could happen in our lives. Having a disabled child had seemed like an incomprehensible tragedy for a mother, especially for a mother like me, who understood nothing of the wonders God had sent her.

I had no idea then just how much joy and light this baby would bring into our lives. I still regret not being able to see that light back then. I was in the middle of the light and still I was blind to it. What a terrible and sad thing....

13

Anthony's Dilemma

THE DAYS passed, amazingly fast.

Maria, our eldest daughter was three, Anthony was two and Nektarios was only one month old. I was breastfeeding him and rocking him almost continually. In fact, even though Anthony was almost two, I was still breastfeeding him too, after all my attempts to wean had failed. Fatigue overwhelmed me, especially at night, but I did not give up. I was obsessed with breastfeeding him. Nektarios would fall asleep only if he was rocked on my legs. He would smile each time I sang to him "Rejoice Nektarios, St. Nektarios." I don't know what connection he made in his mind, but he always smiled at that verse.

Meanwhile, our lives had turned from the dark night back into daylight. Once, while I sang to Nektarios and nursed him with fervor, Anthony came to me with tousled hair, big eyes and a red face, asking me with much agitation, "Mommy, Mommy, tell me, tell me …"

"What is it, my baby?" I asked anxiously, instinctively putting my palm on his forehead, to check if he had a fever.

"Are you feeling sick, my angel?"

I put Nektarios on the pillow and went to Anthony, taking him in my arms. It was 1 a.m., and a full moon was shining in the sky. He looked straight into my eyes with his mysterious long lashes, and asked me, "Mommy, why can't the cow give goat milk?"

I was speechless. My eyes remained fixed on the window. My face looked puzzled. Time froze. I didn't know how to respond. He looked at me so avidly, as if his life depended on my response. I held him tight. Suddenly I burst into tears. I laughed and cried at the same time.

"Let me tell you a story instead, my angel." He didn't seem too happy with my answer, but he obeyed. I held them both in my arms.

I rocked them, I sang to them, and I thought about how happy I was. I was a mother who held on one arm a disabled child who was happy and smiling when I sang to him about St. Nektarios, and, on my other arm, I held another child with serious, dark eyes and long eyelashes, who over the years would ask me thousands of difficult questions, to which I would not always know the answer....

A disabled child on my left arm and a thoughtful child on the right one. I looked at my daughter, Maria, who suddenly started to cry from her bed. I put her on a big pillow and rocked them all. Immediately, all three fell asleep. In fact all four—there was one in my belly. I had found out three days before. I was surrounded by angels. One on the pillow, two in my arms, and one in my belly. I looked out the window—it was such a bright night!

It was as if the moon wanted to tell me a story. My gaze remained fixed somewhere in the night outside. I could not fall asleep. And yet, why can't the cow give goat milk?

14

About Macrina

"Oh my God! I can't, I can't!" I screamed, while the contractions became more violent.... My belly was huge, the largest of all my pregnancies.

I was panting harder and harder.

"My love!" I called to my husband in a supreme panic. I did not want to give birth in front of three children, in the middle of our garden.

My husband was five trees away, playing chess with a neighbor.

"The baby is coming out! I can't hold it anymore! Take me to the hospital quickly," I cried, agitated.

"Wait a bit, my love," my husband answered calmly. "Look, I'm a few moves away from winning."

I looked at him in shock. He was concentrated entirely on the chessboard. He didn't even get off his chair. His entire world, life, dreams were in that game of chess. I felt like taking the board and breaking it over his head. I sat down next to a tree and I watched him as he carried on playing.

Finally, he realized the seriousness of the situation and got off his chair. Grudgingly, he left his game unfinished and put the children and me in the car, and we all went to the hospital.

There, Dr. Raluca, the most sacrificial doctor I had seen in my life, was already waiting for me.

She led me quickly to a delivery room, where obviously I would start with my usual shouts. In the same room, there was another woman in labor, and her presence made me feel terribly embarrassed and ashamed of myself.

She had been told that her baby was already dead, and she was trying to give birth with pain not only in her body, but in her soul as well. At least, despite all the excruciating pain, I knew I was bringing a child to life, while she knew that her baby was dead already. I felt so sad for her!

The doctor held my hand, hugged me, kissed me on my forehead, encouraged me. What wouldn't she do to ease my suffering?

After twelve hours I was still in labor. I felt as if my heart had no more power to beat. "My heart will stop beating!" I screamed to the doctor.

"Either we both die or neither of us. Come on, hang in there!" her answer came.

I looked at her through tears and unimaginable pain. She was so brave. However, I could not give birth.

I was slowly losing consciousness. I felt transparent and light, as if floating to the ceiling.

I heard some quick steps, and another doctor came in and touched my belly. I heard him saying very agitatedly to my doctor, "The baby will break every bone in her. Do something, because otherwise she and the child will die!"

Those creepy words brought me back to reality. Meanwhile, the dead baby was delivered and his mother was so devastated. I saw how her dead baby was put on her chest and she let out the scream of a slaughtered animal. I had not heard a more terrible scream in my life. A howl of almost cosmic pain ...

Her pain filled the room. It had almost become material. The suffering in that delivery room was so thick that one could cut pieces out of it....

"My beautiful baby boy ..." she cried, looking at the baby, holding him to her chest with immense despair. Some nurses wanted to take the baby from her arms, but she did not want to give him up.

"My baby has to be alive," I kept repeating to myself. The pain of giving birth to a dead child seemed unimaginable, impossible to live with. I knew that, when coming out of my belly, my child had to cry, to scream, to give a sign of life. I felt so selfish. That woman was looking at me and, through my almost continuous screams, I caught her look once. It was one of endless sadness, discouragement and despair. I turned my eyes quickly. I could not bear her look.

Compassion for this woman almost left me breathless. Suddenly, somewhere between dream and reality, between nightmare and hope, somehow I managed with a final scream to push the baby out, toward light, toward life. I heard the doctor shouting, "Someone come and help me! It's a heavy child. I can't hold her!"

I froze. "Another disabled child," I thought. "Have mercy on me, my Lord!" was all I could say before I fainted.

A little while later, on my chest was laid a gorgeous girl,

weighing 5.2 kilos.[1] But above all, she was a perfectly healthy child. I could not believe it. I was afraid to be happy. I kept asking, "Are you sure she has no anomaly?" I left the room drunk with happiness.

That other woman was still there, but I couldn't say anything to her. Even now, after so many years, I still blame myself for being a scoundrel.

In that delivery room, death and life had joined hands in a mad dance. Three days later, I left the hospital with a heavy but perfectly healthy baby and with my soul heavy with happiness.

A few months later, two lines appeared on my pregnancy test. "I'm pregnant again, my love" I called to my husband, who was chopping some wood outside. He threw away the ax and took me in his arms with overwhelming joy.

But I had a grim premonition, or perhaps I was extremely tired. I was very scared, with a fear that was going to stay with me throughout my pregnancy. I felt my body could not cope with another labor. After nine months, on November 9, the feast of St. Nektarios, the contractions started. I was rejecting them. I felt I could not take them anymore. Still, on that beautiful night I would give birth to ...

---

[1] About 11.4 pounds.

15

Justina, the One with Dimples

This time, Dr. Raluca was not in the country, so I went to give birth at a hospital in Bucharest, without knowing anyone there.

I had no gift for the doctor. All I had with me was a large icon of the Theotokos. I gave it to the doctor, begging her to do something to help me. I could not breathe. As soon as the icon was in the doctor's hands, the situation changed completely.

I was immediately taken to the operating block, where I had a C-section. They gave me a local anesthesia and from that moment on, everything seemed so surreal. I continually spoke about my four little children at home, while my baby was taken out of my belly incredibly quickly and painlessly. I was desperately waiting to hear the baby's first scream.

Oh boy—when that scream came out of her little lungs, it seemed as if it shattered all the windows and walls of the hospital. A sweet and healthy girl of 3.8 kilos[1] was put on my chest. I was forty-one when I had my fifth child. The fifth miracle of my life. I never knew how to enjoy life as I should. To live with true Christian joy.

---

[1] About 8.4 pounds.

I gave birth to five children in six and a half years. Five different deliveries, one after another, after unimaginably long labors. If I hadn't died during any of my deliveries, then I was to live. To live happily with my five little children, whom I breastfed and loved more than anything. At night, while putting them to sleep, or rocking and nursing them, I counted them, and they seemed like the little dwarves of the forest. They were all so small and sweet. I watched all five of them every night and I caressed them while the babies were sucking all the milk out of me, with an incredible appetite.

They seemed to me from a different world, an eternal world, a world that had been gifted to me. I was holding all of them at my chest, as if they belonged to me only. They were all mine. I think I loved them more than I loved God. I no longer knew where the line was. I didn't know where to stand....

I was vibrating. I was in a state of tension and strain most of the time. An incomprehensible chill was still inside me, a fear without a clear object. It became almost existential. I was to find the reason almost a year and a half later. Then, my life would take a completely new path. Then, my real life would begin. A life lived on the edge, a life lived with maximum intensity. A life tasting of poison ...

16

The Supremacy of the Lump

"WHAT CAN this be, my love?" I asked my husband while, shocked, I felt my left breast. A huge lump of nearly four centimeters appeared in my breast, bursting with an uncontrollable vitality. I was seven months pregnant with Justina.

"Don't worry, my love," my husband reassured me calmly, "Probably just the pregnancy hormones. We'll put a cabbage leaf on it to make it pull back."

"It'll be okay for sure," I said with a frozen smile, trying to reassure him more than myself.

The pains started shortly after. For over a year and a half, from that day until I gave birth, and then for as long as I breastfed Justina, the cabbage leaves became almost one with my being. No day passed without my wrapping them over my breasts, neck, back, and arm. It was as if my brain itself became a huge cabbage. When I closed my eyes, all I could see was cabbage. Sometimes I had violent pains in my left breast. Viorel bought me a mechanical breast pump. Using it made me scream with pain. I didn't know that it would hurt so badly, but I didn't give up. I was fighting for each drop of milk. To me, that milk had become synonymous with life.

I remember how one night my husband brought a car full

of firewood. He was carrying it with his Logan.¹ At 11 p.m., I went out to help him unload the car. The children were asleep. That night I had put them all in the same bed and covered them with a large blanket. Only their little heads could be seen, sweet, plump, and curly. They seemed so many. They filled the whole bed, and the peace and tranquility on their little faces made me feel like heaven was in that room. I went outside, hurried and tense. I started to carry wood, thick and solid wood, real wood, as real as my breast lump. Then, a huge piece of wood fell on my foot. The pain was sharp and quite intense. And then, suddenly, an idea flashed in my mind.

"Maybe the lump will disappear," I said and started to pick up a lot of wood in my arms, so much that I managed to press quite hard against my breast with a huge piece of wood. The pain became unthinkable, but I didn't care. I wanted that wood to hit me so hard, to crush my lump completely. I pressed and pressed with that piece of wood against my breast, in a desperate attempt to make the lump disappear. I would have crushed it in a second. The pain of that blow made my brain explode.

Lord, I kept that wood pressed against my chest and I hit the lump with it in the dark summer night, hit it repeatedly, as if my life and the lives of my little children depended on those blows.

Through tears and groans of pain, all I could see in my mind was the image of my five little children, all sleeping under the blanket, with their little angelic faces, while their

---

[1] A model of Romanian car, made by the manufacturer Dacia.

mother refused to accept the cruel reality: that she might have cancer.

"It is not possible, not possible" I cried. "I have breastfed almost continually for the last seven years."

And I was hitting, hitting with that concrete and real piece of wood against a breast with a lump just as concrete and real. The world, the stars, the whole sky suddenly disintegrated, and I was somewhere outside time and space, with only my bruised breast and my fear. A terrible, petrifying fear.

Finally, my husband found me on my knees, holding a huge piece of wood in my arms, overwhelmed with pain.

"It's still there, it's still there," I cried, sobbing. "It doesn't want to leave, I can't destroy it. Don't you understand?"

"What's still there?" he asked, horrified.

"The lump, that cursed lump …"

He took the piece wood from my arms and took me inside the house, almost carrying me in his arms.

The night had become so heavy and overpowering.

I sat on the bed next to my little children, and I fell asleep, curled next to them like wounded animal. I squatted at their feet and hugged them.

I was tired, so tired …

Suddenly, I felt cold, so cold that my teeth started chattering. Or maybe I was not shivering from cold, but from fear. A fear was flooding my being. A fear that would be part of me as of that moment.

That night, I knew a part of me had died. It was completely, permanently, undeniably gone. From then on, another being was born in me, one for whom I felt total repulsion. That fear would reveal everything uncivil, primitive in me. Overnight I became a coward, a scared and frightened woman. I was frightened of everything and anything. It was as if I were cut in half.

A knife split my being, and what was more, it split my faith.

I could no longer find a support point. Or maybe I had never really had one.

17

The Defeat of the Tumor's Guardian

AFTER A YEAR and eight months of fears, hopes, uncertainties and endless nights of breastfeeding, after refusing with our whole beings to accept the inescapable, Viorel and I finally decided to see a doctor. We went to Pucioasa, to see Dr. Raluca. As soon as we went in her office, I asked her bluntly, "Am I going to die?" and without waiting for her to answer, I showed her the lump on my breast and underarm.

She looked at me shocked. She examined me gently, as if she could not believe her eyes.

"Why did you wait so long?" She did not wait for a reply and started to write a prescription angrily. Her face was extremely pale.

"It can't be that bad," I said to myself, forcing myself to smile and trying to put a brave face on it, but it was all for show. A very low quality show, for that matter.

"Tomorrow, we'll meet urgently at the Military Hospital. I'll introduce you to a professor."

No further explanations were needed. I realized that.

The fact was that never in my life had I felt more stupid....

I felt that I was the definition of stupidity.[1] The next morning we went to the Military Hospital, and Dr. Raluca, paler than ever, introduced us to a Professor Doctor.

After the examination, we were alone in the consultation room with Dr. Raluca seated in front of us. I remember that everything in the room was white, an overwhelming, sparkling white. But it felt oppressive, almost suffocating. For me it was worse than in that latrine where I had fallen when I was seven. I sat in front of her, on a rolling office chair, with my hands clenched tightly to it, because I felt I would collapse any second. That devastating cold gripped me again.

God, how I was shaking!

"Save me for Maria!" I begged her with a strangled voice. I knew she dearly loved my oldest child, Maria, the one with gray eyes at birth....

"We need a biopsy urgently," murmured that angel of a woman.

I kept trembling, trying hard not to fall off the chair.

I was so ashamed that I could not control the terrible trembling that had overtaken me.

Suddenly, I remembered that my husband was somewhere behind me, but I could hardly feel his presence. I turned to him. His face had become almost blue, and he only managed to whisper, "My love ... I no longer feel my hands."

I looked at them. They had lost all color. I took him

---

[1] The self-deprecatory irony of the chapter's title is apparent by this point: In holding off for twenty months before showing the tumor to a doctor, the author had been, as it were, the "tumor's guardian" or protector—and this medical examination was her "defeat."

immediately out in the hallway, and I almost forced him to lie down on a bed, while I began to fervently rub his hands, cheeks, and chest.

"We'll hold on, my love. It'll be okay, we'll fight. Christ, our Savior, won't leave us."

After he was back on his feet, as we hugged with a terrible despair, we stumbled and both fell down on our knees, chained together in an endless pain....

We burst into tears while I kept whispering, "It'll be okay, it'll be okay ..." like an old, forgotten refrain....

The white of the hospital had faded completely. It became a dark gray.

We finally left, holding tightly to each other.

He was holding my hand so tightly, our shoulders were so close. I knew why he did not let go of my hand: he didn't want death to enter between us, didn't want to let it make its way between us.

We left behind that snow-white room, that hospital where my fight with death would begin much sooner than I expected. A somewhat uneven and unfair fight, but a fight which helped me to find out, in the end, the meaning of love.

It was as if I had lived until then for nothing, and only then was I born and saw my true self, a self that I disliked completely. But there was nothing to do; it was mine and I had to accept myself as I was.... Too bad—I understood this too late, perhaps too late for my children.

18

The Shot

THE NEXT DAY we came to the emergency room of a hospital for infectious diseases.

"Excuse me, I came for a biopsy," I said shyly.

"One second," a tall, good-looking doctor replied promptly. "Let me get a gun and I'll sort you out immediately."

Initially, I thought that I had not heard well, but then I realized that the breast had to be "shot" in a certain place, to be more or less hacked. That was the method.

The young doctor left in a hurry, and Viorel and I, almost resigned, waited on a bench in the hospital hallway. Meanwhile, another young doctor appeared, just as good-looking and efficient as the first one. He inquired about our problem, and when he heard I was there for biopsy, he quickly assured us that he would "shoot me in no time" and then rushed down the hallway to get hold of the biopsy gun.

Meanwhile, the first doctor appeared with the (in)famous gun in his hand and invited me solemnly into the consultation room.

I remember that it was during Great Lent, specifically on Holy Friday. Before I had time to get undressed, the second doctor appeared, and he had a rather lively quarrel with the first one, about who was to "shoot" me:

"I saw her first, so I get to shoot her!"

"But today it's my turn, and I don't see why you have to shoot them all," the second doctor promptly replied. It was all so awkward, even pathetic, and I felt a terrible pity for the two of them.

I wished I could tear my shirt off and let them both shoot me.

I was sorry for them in a way. I knew that the unwritten rule was to give some money to the one performing the biopsy. On the other hand, I also felt a little flattered that two young men were fighting over which one of them would "shoot" my breast.

Finally, the situation was resolved peacefully and I, lying on the bed, braced myself for the shot. The pain was so sharp after the first shot that it took my breath away. I tried a forced smile, clutching my hands firmly to the bedside. At the second shot, I bit my lips so hard that they instantly began to bleed. I set my eyes somewhere out the window, and I saw, out of the blue, a little sparrow sitting on a tree branch by the window. While tissue was taken from my breast, I kept looking at that little bird. The sparrow looked back at me with so much compassion, as though she wanted to take away my pain. It was as if there were a bridge between us, a bridge of love. I felt as if the good God had sent that sparrow to strengthen me.

I anchored my eyes on that sparrow. Finally, the shots ended, the pain stopped, the sparrow flew somewhere into the sky, and I left the hospital somehow calmer. In a few days, I was to find out whether I had cancer or not. In two days it would be the Resurrection of the Lord. But nothing resurrected in me. To resurrect, I had to realize something first: the hell within me. I knew that my fight would be primarily with that hell that lay deep inside me, and only then with cancer.

19

Ruthless Malignant Cells

NOT TOO LONG afterwards, we went to the hospital to find out the result of the biopsy. I waited with Viorel for the result, in a line, in a dark hallway. Besides us, there were eight nervous women, waiting for their sentence. My husband held my hand tightly.

Our palms were sweaty from emotion and we were extremely anxious. We did not speak and I kept smiling stupidly, hoping to encourage him somehow. I could not stand still. I walked hectically from one end to the other of the hallway. My knees shook uncontrollably, as if I were connected to an electrical outlet. My thoughts were flying chaotically. I could not pray. I could not concentrate on anything. All I could think of were my little children, with their innocent faces, curly hair, big eyes, and clear smiles. When I thought again of their ages, I felt a despair overtaking me: two, four, five, seven, and almost eight years old.

All still very young.... How to explain this to them ... how to make them understand?

"Mrs. Grigore?" I heard my name called by the doctor.

She invited me into her office. It was like heading toward

a gas chamber. I had no air, and that cold, which had become like second nature to me, engulfed me again.

"I am sorry to inform you, but the cells are malignant. You have cancer."

The diagnosis fell as sharp as an axe.

"Stage 3B."

While she said it, she avoided looking into my eyes. I tried to look into her eyes. I wanted to find a shred of hope in her eyes.

"Are you sure of that? You know, I had been breastfeeding continually for seven years.... Maybe it's a mistake, maybe it's not true ..."

"Madam, it's certain: you have cancer. There's no room for interpretation. I'm sorry."

As we left her office, the lack of air became increasingly acute. We left that dark and cold hallway in a hurry and ran down the stairs without a particular aim.... My husband did not let go of my hand. He held me tight, afraid I would do who knows what.

We stopped in a tiny park in the hospital courtyard. We did not speak. We did not know what to say.

We sat on the grass, leaning against an old tree. Then, I remembered the fall into that latrine when I was seven.

That struggle was reflected in this struggle. I was struggling for air no longer in a mountain of sewage, but in a mountain of helplessness and fear. It was definitely worse than sewage.

"What will I do, my Lord? What am I going to do with five little children, one of them disabled, a sick mother, and blind a mother-in-law?"

I was lost. I looked at the trees in front of me.... I could not meet Viorel's eyes—we both would have burst into tears.

"I know what we need to do," I told my husband as if suddenly awakened from a nightmare. "Let's go to St. Nektarios."[1]

Viorel drove like a madman on the busy streets of Bucharest. He wanted to reach St. Nektarios with the speed of light.[2] Neither of us had patience.

We arrived in front of the relics of the saint. The priest who was there, after I told him that I had cancer, responded promptly and unequivocally:

"The illness is mainly here!" and he pointed with his finger at his temple. "It is primarily in the mind. Struggle must first take place there."

I went to talk to the saint. I didn't tell him anything about me. My brain was somewhat numbed by the prospect of my imminent death. I could not cry. So I just told him how many children I had, how old they were, what each of them liked, how they played, and how they couldn't sleep at night unless we were all embraced in the same bed. I told him how my youngest would hold my face in her hands and how she would calm down when she felt my head in her hands. Like she was weighing it every time.

"St. Nektarios, these are my children, and I beg you to have mercy on them."

On the way back the silence between Viorel and me

---

[1] St. Nektarios is especially considered to be a great intercessor for people suffering from cancer. Many pray before his holy relics for help.

[2] That is, to reach the church of the Radu Vodă Monastery in Bucharest, where part of the saint's relics are kept.

became like a latent bomb. I wished I could cry, howl, and somehow externalize the pain inside. But I had no time for wailing. Five little children, a sick mother, and my husband's blind mother, who were both living with us, waited for me at home. I had to talk to them and make them understand. Understand what? I had no idea yet.

20

The Futility of an Explanation

"My darlings!" I cried when we got home. All five of them ran toward me with incredible speed. They wrapped their arms around my neck, my waist, bit me, pulled me by the hair, kissed me on the lips and cheeks. We hugged almost desperately for a long time. We all went to the bedroom, where my mother was sitting on the bed with her hands in her lap, waiting for me to bring the results. She was so beautiful. She was seventy-eight, pale and slender, with big blue eyes and with her white hair braided in two pigtails at the back. She looked like a picture from a fairy-tale book. Even though my soul was torn into thousands of pieces, I felt I had to tell them. I needed to.

"My darlings, Mommy has a something on her breast. They will give me some injections, and then Mommy will throw up a little, but later she'll be all right."

"Enough of that," promptly said Maria, my eldest daughter, who was seven. "Just tell me if you're going to die."

"No, my love, it's just that things will be a little difficult for a while, but everything will be okay."

Macrina and Justina, my younger girls, both of them with blond hair and green eyes, who were only four and two, jumped into my arms and started to caress my breast. They were caressing precisely the one with the tumor. And it felt like the tumor was shrinking under their little hands.

God, how I wanted it to miraculously go away! I made a sign to my husband to take the children out of the room. Without looking into my mother's eyes, I told her abruptly, "I have cancer." Just as abruptly she stood up and went outside to get some fresh air. She was crushed by the news. I wanted to hug her, but I could not. I would be crushed by a mountain of pain. I went quickly to the kitchen and started mechanically to do some dishes. It was only later that I realized that they were clean to begin with, but I just needed to do something, so I carried on. At some point, tired, I sat on the bed in the kitchen.[1] I was so tired that I could barely breathe. It wasn't a physical fatigue, but a metaphysical tiredness. It felt as if I hadn't slept for a thousand years.

I lay on the bed wishing only to fall asleep, as quickly and for as long as possible. I wished for an endless sleep.

I hadn't even started the fight and I was ready to give up. The thought gave me chills.

If I was not able to fight … then my children …

Hopelessness flooded my heart. I recognized the feeling—it was the same awful feeling I had had in the hospital courtyard, after the birth of Nektarios.

I started to feel cold, as a terrible despair and fear took over me. Viorel, my husband with the name of a flower,[2] came in and knelt at my side, took my hands in his hands, rough

---

[1] Romanian country houses usually have a bed in the kitchen.

[2] The name Viorel is derived from the *vioreaua* (*Scilla bifolia*, or alpine squill) plant, the flowers of which are usually deep violet-blue.

from labor, and begged me with the gentlest voice in the world, "My love, will you promise me that you'll fight? I beg you to fight! Don't leave me alone with five little children. I can't live without you, don't you understand? I love you!"

He almost squashed me with his embrace. All of a sudden, our meager kitchen had become a beautiful, surreal palace, and my husband was the most wonderful prince. Even the cold in my bones melted away like magic.

"I'll fight, my love! I'll fight! I promise!"

Suddenly we both broke into a liberating sob. I had never felt his love in such a tangible and real way. He seemed the safest and most steadfast rock I could hold onto.

That night we all slept in one bed, with five little pairs of hands and feet all over us. We were so happy we were together. We were so happy to be still alive. I watched them sleep. And I noticed that my husband had suddenly gone gray.

All night I kissed their feet and the hands of my husband. They seemed to belong entirely to me. I thought they were mine, that I deserved them. Their lives depended on me. Their happiness was inseparable from my happiness.

I was so mistaken.... Nothing was mine.... Neither them, nor their lives, nor even my life was my own. Only fear was mine.

I finally fell asleep after an extremely difficult battle with myself. I was about to start a war in which I would lose so many battles that I would lose count. But no matter how ravaged, wounded, bloody or poisoned I was going to be, I had to stay alive for a little longer; my five little children had to have their mother with them.

"Mother of God, have mercy on them, I beg you!"

That was all I could say, and I kept repeating it hundreds of times.

The next morning I went again to the hospital. There I was about to meet some people who seemed to be sent from heaven. People who showed me that there was something more valuable than our own lives: sacrifice for the other.

I had not thought life could be as intense as I felt in that hospital.

Meeting the director of the "Rebirth Foundation," which functioned within the hospital, had a great impact on me. The name of the foundation was not accidental. Many lives were saved through its programs. At least those with early-stage cancer.

I saw her coming toward me. A tall, redheaded, good-looking woman, with a large and sincere smile. She was bursting with optimism.

"Madam, I am a mother. I have five little children. Please tell me openly, from a medical point of view, do I have any chance? Otherwise, I must find a mother for my five children." I kept talking to her, strangled with emotion.

My husband also jumped in almost incoherently, "Madam, I cannot live without my wife and, if necessary, I will sell the house, my kidneys, I will sell everything only to save her...."

She looked at us with a rare understanding. She kept encouraging and hugging us, while she showed us into a small room. There she introduced us to a lady doctor who would disturb my life, make it a mess, poison it, and prolong it at the same time.

21
Death- and Life-Giving Chemo

THE DOCTOR was an incredibly beautiful young woman. She was young: thirty, maybe forty. She reminded me of Elizabeth Taylor in her heyday, with her black hair and green eyes.

She seemed so young, and I couldn't help wondering when she had had time to learn so much.

"Please tell me, should I start looking for another wife for my husband? I have to know whom he will marry.... You see, I have five little children and I need to leave them in good hands. I don't want a stepmother who would beat them every day."

My question left her speechless. I strongly believed in what I was saying. I didn't care if she thought I was crazy.

She calmly felt my breast. She smiled lightly and told me that she would let me know when I should start seeking a new wife for my husband.

She wrote a prescription and sent me for blood tests. She did not say much. Before leaving the room, I looked at her, trying to catch a sign, a little hope, anything. But she was impenetrable. Confused, I left. After a few days I went back to the hospital to start the drip, the famous "red" drip, which would leak poison into my veins. It was the life-giving and death-giving poison called Tamoxifen, a name that brought to my mind the Italian Mafia. I imagined Al Capone shooting me in broad daylight in the hospital's hallway. I lay on the bed, with my husband beside me, holding my hand tightly, while the drip began to poison me slowly. The poison would kill and prolong my life at the same time. In fact it would prolong a life of agony, a false life, but I did not care. My five children had to have me with them a little while longer.

After six hours, I got up from the bed and I was quite amazed at how well my body had handled the first chemo. When I tried to walk toward my husband I suddenly felt drunk. The ceiling, the walls, the windows—everything was spinning around me in a crazy dance. However, it was quite okay. I was expecting something much worse, much more dramatic.

"Aren't you proud of me, my love?" I asked my husband "Look how well I cope."

He shook my hands with power as if he were awarding me some kind of medal of honor, and we went home with our hopes high.

"Mommy, Mommy, we're so glad you're back!" My children hugged me with unspeakable joy.

We kissed, we pinched, we tickled. I could not believe it.... I was with my angels, and all I could feel after the chemo was a slight dizziness and confusion, as if I had drunk barrels of wine. But when I was most proud of my body's resistance, suddenly jets of vomit splashed out of me like a fountain.

But I was not vomiting normally; it was coming out of me

with an incredible force, and I could not control it at all, as if something in my body had exploded.

The children, somewhat horrified by what they saw, scattered everywhere.

Maria ran to me with a bucket, Anthony with a towel. Macrina quickly tried to draw something on a piece of paper, and Justina screamed for her father, "Daddy, Daddy—Mommy is leaking and she won't stop!"

Eventually it stopped. I calmed down and washed myself. I had a look in the bathroom mirror and I was in for another shock: brown spots of various sizes had appeared on my hands, face, legs, and shoulders. Everything seemed out of control. Just then, Anthony came in carrying a huge encyclopedia and told me excitedly, "Mom, did you know that cockroaches can survive for a whole week without their head?"

I looked at him horrified. I had a pathological fear of them, and if I saw one, I would simply start screaming.

Given the state I was in, this wasn't exactly the best possible timing for receiving this piece of information.

"Really, my love? A whole week without their head?"

I tried to look interested in what he was saying, mostly not to disappoint him.

"Yes, Mom, imagine that!"

His eyes shone with excitement; those terribly long eyelashes were blinking frantically. Whenever he discovered something, he got so excited, as if he had just discovered the wheel or fire or something like that. Considering how bad I was, imagining a headless cockroach crawling threateningly toward me and climbing slowly up my leg toward my heart, toward my eyes—it was too much. It was worse than the chemo itself.

That night my husband squeezed countless kilos of lemons and oranges. My sickness was inhuman, total, and devastating.

I had not imagined that the sickness could be so overwhelming. The next day we went again to the hospital. I was covered in brown spots, and the doctor, calm and confident, gave me some allergy pills.

"It will be okay," she reassured me, and we went home.

It was a long and tiring journey back home. Our home, where five little children were waiting for me, full of excitement and hope. There, I could breathe their love, their innocence, their power to make me smile, their strength to fight alongside me. To keep me alive.

22

Life-Saving Biochemistry

OVER THE MONTHS, I was surprised to discover what huge and fantastic power the human body has to regenerate. It was terrible: every three weeks I would give blood—not once but dozens, hundreds of times—and then I would receive a drip, in accordance with the test results.

I watched how the blood was taken from me with inescapable regularity.

Every three weeks I watched with amazement how my body fought resolutely against death and against the chemotherapy itself.

I was sorry that I could not learn from my body's perseverance, ambition, strength, and despair to stay alive. It was like an out-of-body experience every time. As if my body, my brain, were fighting somehow autonomously—as if someone else inside me were ready to fight and to make any sacrifice to keep me alive.

I felt somewhat limp, with no will left in me. I would leave myself at the mercy of my body and its incredible power of regeneration. I was amazed by my own body every time I went for tests.

Every three weeks it was the usual, terrible nausea and

vomiting. I couldn't swallow any food. I was actually glad I could not eat, since I weighed seventy-five kilos,[1] but I was worried that I couldn't even drink water. I threw up everything. At night, my husband woke up with unthinkable regularity and squeezed lemons and oranges. What simply devastated me was that even though we had an electric juicer, he did not want to use it. He only wanted to squeeze the fruits with his hands. I was looking from the other room at his wrinkled, tired hands, straining to get the juice from those fruits, to give some life to my sick and poisoned cells. And not only for a night or two, or ten or a hundred … but a continuous row of nights.… It was as if we had both entered eternity. He was carrying on with a mad desire to resist, to fight, to defeat death, even partially. He entirely changed my perception of what love is. We had been married for almost ten years, but never before had I felt more loved and protected.

Every night I would hear him waking up quietly, and then I would hear, in the heavy silence of the night, the juice dripping into the glass. And if I listened carefully, I would hear life dripping out of me, and the same time his love dripping hope into my veins. The hope that my end had not come and that, with his devotion and sacrifice, he could build around me an impenetrable wall, a wall that death could not breach.

His power of sacrifice was a miracle to me.

I watched him every night, waking up every two hours and bringing me a tall glass of orange and lemon juice. He

---

[1] About a hundred and sixty-five pounds.

always waited for me to drink it to the last drop. He was so sweet ... like a child waiting for a miracle.

And I was so ashamed.... I was ashamed to embrace him because I felt that I smelled like death, like rotting, like the end of life. I was ashamed by his perseverance, an unbreakable perseverance. The next day we started everything all over again. My children begged me to eat but I couldn't get anything down my throat. One morning, Anthony came with a handful of encyclopedias, his eyes shining. I braced myself for whatever information he was about to deliver.

"Mommy! Mommy, you shouldn't whine that you cannot swallow. Listen to this: beginning in 1966, a Frenchman named Michel Lotito ate and digested ten bicycles, seven TV sets, six chandeliers, and a light Cessna aircraft. Do you realize, Mom, how much that man swallowed?"

This piece of information made me not only nauseous but also angry. I was suddenly so irritated with that man who could swallow all those monstrosities, while I could not eat a bowl of soup.

"Mommy, Mommy, let me tell you some more!" My little scientist started to bomb me with information from his encyclopedia.

"Please, my love, just don't tell me who swallowed what, because I'm pretty sure I'll vomit!"

"Mommy, this one is not about that. But did you know that one kilogram of radioactive Uranium-235 could provide the necessary quantity of atomic energy to keep a light bulb lit for 27,400 years.... Can you imagine that?"

I remained quiet, staring at the floor.

"Mommy, aren't you glad that we could have energy for so many thousands of years, and we could survive as a planet?"

Suddenly I realized that I had become selfish. I wasn't interested at all in the survival of the planet. I was only interested in my own survival. My concern and drama was that my little girl, Justina, could not fall asleep unless she held my cheeks with her little hands.

If I suddenly disappeared, where would she find other cheeks, another mother, another motherly love?

I watched her every night as she slept. Blond, with green eyes, with dimples so sweet and deep that it seemed angels nested in them. I watched her searching for my cheeks with her hands and how she found her peace only when she felt them under her fingers. She touched me almost desperately, as if she were measuring my head and then, when she found my cheeks, she smiled happily, revealing those deep dimples. I wished I could turn back time and put her again in my womb, to protect her from all the suffering in the world.

Almost a year passed, twelve months during which Anthony bombarded me with thousands of pieces of information from his encyclopedia, Justina choked me every night with her chubby hands, Maria made up incredibly sad poems, Macrina drew nights with a blue full moon and a meteorite threatening to hit the earth, Nektarios played all the time with my fingers, and my husband squeezed oranges with a perseverance and confidence that I could not classify in any system of values. That year he must have squeezed a mountain of oranges for me. A mountain of oranges squeezed from a sea of love.

23

The Removal

I COULD NOT believe it. I frantically touched my breast and underarm. There was no lump. There was no more agonizing, overwhelming fear of death, of the end, of not being able to hug my children, of not being able to love them like crazy.

"Doctor, there's no lump!" I told him panting, unable to believe my breast might be as it was in the beginning when I was breastfeeding, when I could feel the mouths of my five toddlers desperately sucking my milk. I had never been happier than when I was breastfeeding them. I was amazed at how the breast that had nourished them was the same which was spreading death throughout my body.

I had breastfed for seven years. My left breast had done its duty. Five babies had been fed from it. It seemed impossible to accept that it would be cut off and thrown into a garbage bin.

"We have to cut it off," the doctor said implacably.

I looked at him in shock. I could not understand. I felt so stupid. Why did he have to cut it off if the lump was gone? I looked at him, astonished. He was young and handsome. Tall, dark, with curly hair, he seemed like a handsome American actor from the sixties. He seemed from another time. Next to him was a lady doctor paying close attention to him. She seemed to be a very strong woman. Beautiful, self-confident. She emanated a power of sacrifice and compassion toward all women with breast cancer. She encouraged me a lot. Whenever she entered the room, I smiled, and she always smiled back. To me, those smiles were worth more than a million words.

Although I had been hospitalized for two days and set for surgery, I hadn't unpacked yet, so I started to get my pajamas out of my bag. I was confused and scared. I had been away from my children for only three days, and already I missed them terribly. My tears flowed like a river. I could not hold them back. As I took my night shirt out of my bag, an envelope fell down. I had no idea where it came from. I had packed neither money nor letters.

I rushed to open it. I felt my knees give out and I sat on the bed. Tears flooded my face. I read and I cried … I cried and I read….

"Mommy, my sweet Mommy … I beg you to fight. If you fight, I will live. But if you don't fight, I promise you that I will stop eating and I will follow you to heaven. I love you so much. Maria."

I sat on the bed in a state of shock, with my eyes fixed on a wall. It was the letter of a seven-year-old girl, a child's desperate cry. A child who by a divine miracle happened to be mine. This was my daughter's suffering, the suffering of a seven-year-old girl who could not imagine living without her mother.

I felt like I had been hit by a truck.

My daughter's pain hurt me enormously.

I felt extremely guilty and so terribly sorry that I had not died when I was seven in that latrine, that I had not been covered by that mountain of sewage. It hurt me so that I had survived and given birth to five children who needed their mother so badly. It hurt me so that in the mind and heart of a seven-year-old girl was the idea that, if her mother was gone, she had no reason to live.

I would have gladly done a hundred years of chemotherapy rather than bring so much suffering to my children.

It hurt me so when everyone kept telling me to fight, fight.... I did not know how to fight. I did not know how to think or how to feel. I did not know how to live anymore.

I ran to the bathroom and collapsed on the floor, bursting into tears. It was useless. I wanted to bang my head on the wall. I had made such huge mistakes. All my life, I had never had a breast scan. I had children after the age of thirty-four, and I thought that the simple act of breastfeeding could protect me from cancer.

I wished that none of my children knew of my disease ... but I could not hide it. I tried to hide in the garden, to go behind the house to throw up. I tried to cry in dark rooms or in the basement of our house. But it was impossible to keep it from them. They found me every time and they would wipe away my tears with their small, chubby hands, kissing me, biting me, reviving me, resurrecting me.

The surgery was on a Friday. I was taken by a nurse to the surgery room. We passed through a dark and cold hallway. On the way, I silently begged the Holy Mother of God to go home to my children and cover them with her Holy Protection. I prayed with endless despair.

I kept telling her that I had five children, as if the Holy Mother of God didn't know that.

My thoughts were completely crazy. Even Justina, who was only three, could have prayed more coherently and specifically. I reached the surgery room. My knees were trembling, as if I had drunk gallons of vodka. I lay on a cold bed and looked around, frightened. Everything was white and metallic. The old feeling of cold overwhelmed me again. I was put on an IV and I fell asleep almost instantly. Before falling asleep, just before the ceiling started spinning, I begged the Holy Mother of God once more to go to my home and take care of my children. Strangely, I also gave her the exact address (I must have been completely crazy!). My eyelids got heavier and heavier until they closed like two iron gates. At one point, I heard an extremely loud and sharp noise, as if something metallic had fallen on something else cold and metallic. I sat up suddenly and smiled at the doctors in the room. I was laid back and finally fell asleep again. All I remember was floating and floating, until ...

24

The Flight

I HAD the most fascinating, overwhelming, and surreal experience of my life.

I had read in the Holy Fathers that we should not trust in dreams. I had read and knew that they could be deceitful, but what I felt while in surgery had a coherence, clarity, and brightness that I had never experienced in my life. I was flying, flying to the heights, and I was light as a snowflake, as if I were only spirit, only consciousness. I could see the earth, so beautiful, colored in green and blue.

Lord, what heavenly colors, what bright colors! I felt so light, and nothing hurt me anymore, neither my breast, nor my bones, nor my hands. I felt no nausea, and I did not miss my kids.

It was a different kind of longing, of love. I did not feel that infinite despair of not being able to be with them.

I was so light and quiet, at peace with myself and with everything around me.

After some time, I began to see the clouds, the trees, the houses, and the grass!

The grass and the trees were of an unimaginable green.... I had never seen such a green in my life.... It was a green like at the beginning of the world, the initial green of the world. And I was flying with great ease, and I could see at the same time in front of me, behind me, and on the sides.... I was suddenly in harmony with the trees, the grass, the sky. And, as I flew faster, I became lighter and happier, and I felt submerged in an unspeakable peace.

It was like a grain of peace, but still it engulfed me completely. It was a feeling that I had never felt before, a peace that seemed not to be from the world in which I used to live, a peace that suddenly took away all my bodily pain and instantly annihilated my heart's grief, a grief which was far more painful than the physical pain.

I don't know how long the flight, the joy, and the peace lasted; how long I was given to feel my pains lifted—that peace which no words could ever express, in all its splendor and clarity.

I woke up suddenly in a hospital room with two beds. Next to me was the handsome young doctor. When I looked at him, he seemed paler than I was.

He looked at me, concerned and extremely worried, as if I had returned from the dead....

"Mommy of five little children, you're back!" He smiled and took a deep breath, as if he had been raised from the dead together with me.

He embraced me with care. I was connected to all kinds of drips and wires.

I returned the smile, which was somewhat forced and false, and tried to thank him. I had given them nothing, nothing to him or to the lady doctor, and this made me feel awful.

Nevertheless, I don't think they would have accepted my money. They both came into my life at a very difficult time.

"I don't have the words to thank you ..." And I fell asleep again, longing to experience that flight once more—to feel again so light, so alive. But it didn't happen.

I started the recovery process—terrible painful days, days when I tried to feel my breast that was no longer there. Instead, there was a huge cut, a pump, and some long strands through which blood was flowing: red, black, green, all colors.

I thought that, from then on, I would stop being a complete woman. That from then on, I would stop being a true wife to my husband and, what was the most painful, that I would stop being a complete mother with two breasts.

When I got home, my three-year-old girl, Justina, told me while embracing me sweetly and tenderly, "It's okay, Mommy, we'll pray and another breast will grow."

But it never grew. And ever since, I haven't felt like a complete woman, or a complete soul. One thing, however, remained whole, unaltered, and untouched inside me: the flight—the flying that had given me a taste of heaven for a moment. Or, rather, it had given me peace, the peace that I had been seeking, more or less consciously, my entire life.

I felt I would cut off not only one breast, but a thousand breasts if I had them, only to live again that joy. I had been given a moment of eternity, but I didn't really know how to cherish it.

After a few weeks, that peace and joy seemed so far away, almost gone. Fortunately, there were still times when, on long winter nights, when my whole body ached, when the shadow of my missing breast hurt, I would close my eyes and, through tears of devastating sadness, I would imagine that I flew like I had back then. I wished I had died then. I would have given anything to fly once more, to again feel that peace, but it never happened again.

I was left only with the pain that consumed me in the long sleepless nights, a pain that covered me with its dark agony. And there was the memory of a dream that took me for a moment to heaven, a moment for which I would go through cancer ten or a hundred times again. A flight for which one would gladly die....

25

The MD2 Accelerator

AFTER SURGERY, I was sent to radiation. I had to be irradiated. That's how it had to be. I met the doctor who would be responsible for my irradiation. He had a beard and looked like a character from a Russian novel. He had a commanding baritone voice that imposed distance and respect. At first, I was more scared of him than of the radiation. He stated the risks and asked me how long I thought a session would last. I had no idea. He answered that it was no longer than three minutes. Upon having a look at my medical records and seeing a four-centimeter spot on my liver, he decided to send me for more detailed tests.

I refused categorically. There was no time. I felt this like an unshakable conviction. I came to a huge lobby where, to my amazement, I saw around thirty people waiting in line. After a couple of hours, it was my turn to go inside. The huge, heavy sliding doors closed automatically behind me. I felt a terrible choking sensation. I lay half naked on a bed while a device resembling a small-scale spacecraft was placed above my breast. It started to tick. I could tell that each tick was partly life and partly death. For three minutes, I silently cried a prayer to all the saints I knew. The ticking came to an end, and so did the intensity of my prayer.

I sighed with relief when those huge, heavy metal doors opened. Dozens and dozens of times I would pass through them, in and out, and every time I had the horrible feeling that they would not open to let me out.

I was irradiated in the evening. Every evening I went with all my children to the hospital, where they would try to prolong the agony of my life, a life that seemed to me more and more useless. Radiation was tiring. I had no strength to take care of my children or to cook for them.

There wasn't any meal waiting for them when they came home from school or from kindergarten.

I needed a full day to make a soup. When it was ready, it was a victory, as if I had climbed Everest. I would start cutting the vegetables at 9 a.m., and only four hours later would the soup be ready.

My body would shake so hard, even when I lay in bed. I would turn off the stove a few times, and would lie in bed and cry. They were probably tears of pride.

I had been a fast, agile, tireless wife and mother. "My real woman," my husband used to call me. Now, I was holding onto tables and chairs when I walked in the house, and I sat wherever I could. I could not control my heartbeats. Most of the time, I felt like something was about to explode in my head. But what hurt the most was that I was tiring my children every night with that long and grueling trip to the hospital in Bucharest. And once we were there, we had to wait for hours in order for me to go in for three minutes. But many times we were told that the machine wasn't working because it had overheated, and we were simply sent back home.

I remember that one night we were once again in front of the closed doors, and the machine refused to work. A janitor with a bucket in his hand passed by us. I was so crazy with waiting that I asked—rhetorically of course—if they could cool down that confounded machine with some buckets of water. It was as if, only when it was my turn to go in, or just after the doors had closed behind me, the reactor no longer wanted to tick. Dozens of patients in the lobby were crazy from so much waiting.

It was as if the unsettledness inside me interfered with the reactor, causing it to stop working. But that night—a deep and frosty night—I told my husband, being very annoyed, "This is why I married an engineer. Go this instant and repair that reactor, because I can't stand it anymore."

My husband, with the air of a Harvard scientist, went to talk to the janitor. A man in overalls came, a Jack-of-all-trades, one you would expect to save the whole planet from an inevitable cataclysm. He tried to explain to my husband something like the third law of thermodynamics.

My husband, like Hamlet in his great existential dilemma, asked him why the reactor got overheated and why there was no water for its cooling system. The man, in a state of awe, looked up, pointing with his finger above his head, as if saying that it was the management's rules. My husband didn't give up, arguing that a European hospital should never be left without water, electricity, or oxygen. Then the discussion became too technical, and I could only catch words such as buffer, auxiliary system, fire safety.... Then the man suddenly cheered up and concluded triumphantly, "It's the water! I'll go see what I can do."

Even my three-year-old daughter, Justina, would have figured out it must have been the water. However, the reactor did not want to work that night. We left around 11 p.m., unsuccessful, tired, angry and exhausted. On our way back, the stars seemed like lanterns that lit the way. The children were asleep in the back of the car. At some point, my husband overtook another car. After a few minutes, we noticed that car chasing us, overtaking our car, and then it stopped suddenly, blocking our way. My husband braked abruptly. A fierce man got out the other car, with a baseball bat in his hands, and started to hit our car with a rain of blows. The children woke up and started to scream. There was a general chaos. Under the rain of curses and blows, my husband wanted to go outside and fight back. I held him with all my strength. I screamed hysterically, telling him that outside were three more men and he was alone.

"I beg you, let's go!" I cried desperately.

He managed to slip by the other car with great skill and started accelerating more and more.

The car with the men with bats chased us, following us closely. It was getting closer and closer. The other car was like my cancer. The closer it got, the stronger and more devastating it seemed. The distance became smaller, and the children looked back terrified. The other car's headlights almost blinded us. Their hatred and anger was devastating. Viorel sped up and we managed to lose the attackers in the dark night. We finally stopped the car and I went to the back to hug and comfort the children. Anthony, our six-year-old boy, was trembling the most, and told me through tears and hiccups, "Mommy, Mommy, they hit us fourteen times with the bat, eighteen times with their feet, and nine with their fists." I knew he liked math, but not that much. At home, we slept again, embracing, all in the same bed, as if not wanting to be separated by any speeding cars or aggressive men, or even by death.

I fell asleep, looking out the window at the stars, silently thanking God that we were still alive, that we could still sleep all together, and especially that we still felt that sense of security given by "home."

"Glory to Thee, O Lord, glory to Thee!" I got to say once, and I fell into a heavy and deep sleep.

26

The Irradiation of Yesterday, Today, and Tomorrow

THE SAME nightmare almost every night ... And when I say nightmare, I mean primarily for my children. The trip was very tiring. A two-hour trip, then a three-hour wait for only three minutes of irradiation. When we got home it was almost midnight. Dozens of nights almost the same, dozens of nights of an extremely tiring routine. I felt like a criminal mother, not a loving one. One evening, loathing my own cowardice and determined to put an end to that long trip towards life and at the same time towards death, I told my husband, "As of now, I will not go to the hospital anymore.... I don't want the childhood of my children to be defined by disease, hospital rooms, and accelerators. That's it! I'm fed up!"

Viorel calmly got all our kids in the car, and then he took my hand and squeezed it until I had tears of pain in my eyes. His almost crazy gesture amazed me more than the pain itself. With his face red and almost trembling, he yelled, "If in one minute you are not in the car, I am not responsible for my actions. I don't know what I will do to you! A thousand, ten thousand nights—if we have to go to the hospital, we will do it.... With five or a hundred children with us, I don't care.... It's important for you to live.... It doesn't matter how.... Poisoned, irradiated, cut ... All that matters is for these kids to see you among them.... Don't you understand? Get in the car!"

I moved automatically. I had tears in my eyes, but I did my best not to cry in front of my children. My husband had never yelled at me before. He had never been violent. His outburst hurt me. But I knew he was doing this out of desperation, or out of love, or out of both at the same time.

And so, we carried on every night ... night after night ... day after day.... Until the reactor stopped ticking and suddenly I escaped from the long and tiring trip, and I suddenly heard only the ticking hearts of my husband and children, and then suddenly I heard only the ticking of life.

God, I was so happy when everything was over! I was not going anywhere anymore with all five kids, and we could play again and stay in the yard until late, on the swing under the trees, and watch the stars and the moon and the planes passing over us. We would sway in the moonlight and I would tell them the story of the Little Prince, and I was thinking that, just like in the famous story, they all tamed me, tamed my fear and my dread and my despair, and it was like their innocence tamed my fear, that terrible fear of not making them suffer because of me, that overwhelming fear of devastating their soul. And then we would all fall asleep on the swing, very crowded but extremely happy, looking at the stars and the planes passing over us.

27

Wonderful Times

I FELT truly alive, as if reborn from my own ashes. I had stopped chemotherapy and radiotherapy, I was not going to any other surgery, and I had no strong pains.

I was alive and well, and my children had a mother.... I was happy beyond measure. All I felt was a terrible fatigue, as if I were a thousand years old. I could not stand for more than two hours before I had to sit down and rest. Fatigue and fear, a fear that insinuated deep into my cells, a primitive fear ... a fear that stopped me from going back to the hospital, even for a summary checkup. Days, weeks, months had passed, and I tried to lie to myself so beautifully. "Everything has passed; I got rid of the cancer," I silently repeated to myself almost every day.

While in the hospital, I had learned what the cancer path was: malignant cells travelling from the breast to the lung, from the lung to the brain, from the brain to the bone, and so on. It was only a matter of time, but I refused to believe it.

I indulged myself in beautiful illusions and thoughts, and I would say to myself, "I have five children; it was all a bad dream; they need me so much...." And so, I went every weekend to Ghighiu Monastery, to the miracle-working icon of the

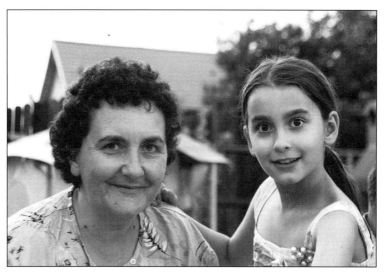

Mioara and Maria, June 16, 2010.

Virgin. It gave me so much hope; she looked at me with such tenderness. I still refused to fight. Deep down I felt that the cancer had not left me, that it was not gone from my being and cells, and that it was a part of me so deeply that it had become practically one with me—we had become consubstantial.

I became a true coward. My whole being revolted: I did not want to know that I had a disease, not to mention an incurable one, although each day my body would tremble as if hit with high voltage, and I would continue to work with an unequalled desperation. I did daily laundry and dishes, washed windows and carpets. I especially liked to wash carpets. When I managed to wash a carpet, I would feel so alive, and everything would seem so real and beautiful. My hair grew back. I felt like a woman loved by her husband again. When he told me I was beautiful, I would blush. I knew he was lying to me, but his lie felt so good.

I remember that one day, on a beautiful autumn afternoon, all five children fell asleep on the swing. I watched them and I could not believe it. My husband said that it was more likely for Halley's Comet to come than for all five kids to be asleep at the same time. Their little faces showed so much tranquility and peace! Viorel was scything the grass in the garden. I was looking at him. He was wearing shorts and he was naked to the waist, with a scythe in his hands, all sweaty and unshaven. I liked him so much when he was growing a beard!

He was the perfect image of the Romanian peasant, descended into my garden from ancient times.... He was the authentic peasant, the true Romanian. I looked at him with so much love and admiration.... I watched him as he scythed, moving the scythe with the precision of a watchmaker, and how the hay lay humble and docile at his feet. I was looking at this man who had fought for hundreds of days for my life, with an inner strength equivalent to dozens of atomic bombs. He took all my fears and infirmities and carried me on his back with a phenomenal desire to keep me alive. A desire much greater even than my own.

He seemed so strong, so desperate, and I was so much in love with him. I remember how that day the whole yard smelled of newly cut hay, the wind blew slightly, and the image of my husband scything was like a picture from a storybook.

It was like reliving the first days of our romance. I went quickly inside, and put on a red dress that he had bought for my birthday. I arranged my hair, which was curly again as he liked it, and with my heart beating fast in my chest, I brought him a pot of buttermilk. He was thirsty. The milk was so cold and he was so hot. I watched him sipping that refreshing milk, with so much appetite. As he drank it, he looked at me with so much love that I felt all adrift. His look and the smell of freshly scythed hay bemused me. He finished drinking and he had milk on his mustache and beard. Trembling, I went closer and wiped away the milk, covering him with kisses. I was so indebted to this man, so grateful to this man who by some miracle was my husband. I didn't know how to thank him. He had prolonged my life with his love. We were both under the trees in the garden that beautiful autumn afternoon, and my husband, my authentic Romanian peasant, hugged me with great force. His embrace almost hurt me. But it was such a sweet pain!

    He threw me on a large bed of leaves and hay, under an old walnut tree, and amidst kisses and hugs he called me "my true woman." He loved me so wildly. We were both sweaty and full of dust, with leaves and hay stuck to our bodies, smelling like peasants and eternity. Those were unforgettable love moments. Time and space no longer existed. Leaves, hay, wind— all nature seemed to merge with us ... as if it were the beginning of the world.... Just him and me, and near us a pot of buttermilk.... And between us, just love, a love that conquered death for a moment, a love that brought me back to life. A life so full and alive, like the red of the dress I was wearing, a life like a gorgeous autumn day, smelling of buttermilk and newly scythed hay.

28

Meeting Supreme Joy

"What if the cancer has not gone from me?" I would ask myself every night.

Dozens, hundreds of nights had passed. As the days passed, I struggled with my fear even more. Cancer could come back sooner or later. Why should I be an exception? I knew I hadn't radically changed my way of thinking, and especially of living. I was still passionate, in love with everything and anything, and especially possessive. I loved my children almost pathologically, as if they were all mine. I knew I was wrong.... I had not learned detachment at all. I was chained, chained to everything and anything; I had never been really free, or maybe I had not yet learned to be free. All my life I had complacently lived in the prison of my own passions. I was not fighting at all to get out of it—or, if I was, I was not doing enough. At first, I would feel something like an impulse, but then I would quit. I would quit before I started the fight to release myself. I had lived my life in chains until I had been thrown into the most overwhelming adventure of my life. An adventure of knowledge, through which I had been given the miracle of meeting some people who would cut the chains that were choking me, people who would try to set me free. What was certain was that I had found a miracle—or, more precisely, I had found joy. The joy of living and especially joy in suffering. I did not think this was possible, and yet …

I was up on the mountain, with our spiritual father. I could not understand how he could love both my husband and me so much. He had and still has so much patience with us. Neither one of us was really doing anything to change for the better. "Patience," he told us, "a little more patience." I did not have much patience; in fact, I do not know if I had ever had any. There were many people at the monastery. I sat on the grass outside and my kids were next to me. That day, I felt such a sadness. It almost solidified in me. I felt a huge weight on my heart, as if that entire mountain were pressing on my heart.

My children were hungry, especially Nektarios, whom I didn't know how to calm down. "Mommy, food, food, Mommy," he repeated all the time. The sermon was almost over. When it was time to say "Our Father," all my five children stretched out their hands to help me stand up. My body was trembling terribly; it was very hot outside, and it seemed that all my cells had gone crazy. After the prayer, I sat heavily back on the grass.

Suddenly, an angelic being appeared in front of me. She was tall, thin, and delicate, as if she had descended directly from heaven. "What beautiful and sweet children you have!" she addressed me in plain Romanian.

"She's human," I said to myself, as for a moment I thought that she was an angel who had come down to earth. I looked at her, dazzled. I was amazed and intrigued by her smile.… Her joy was so sincere.… She seemed so alive. It seemed almost impossible for someone to spread so much joy. As I found out later, she had three little children herself. I thought, "Doesn't she have any financial difficulties or any health issues, or any problems like all of us? What is filling her with so much joy?"

Obviously, the love of Christ; and yet each person has their falls, their invading sorrows.

She seemed to be an exception. She rejoiced almost blatantly. And she almost hit you over the head with her joy.

"Pray for me," I snapped. "You know, I have cancer, but I don't know if it went away or if it went elsewhere, and I'm so afraid to do the tests, to find out, and I have five children."

My eyes filled with tears ready to burst out. I think I looked like a stray dog, alone and sad. Then she suddenly embraced me with a force that effectively disoriented me. "It'll be okay," the angelic being reassured me, all radiant. She had a forceful delicacy rarely seen. Delicate and extremely strong at the same time, that's how she was, that human being I met on a Sunday in the mountains. She would give me a most precious gift. "Come to our church. I'll introduce you to so many wonderful people."

Indeed, she did introduce me to people who would become heroes to me. In fact, my whole life I had always wanted to meet special people and introduce them to my children. When I read them stories at night I wondered, "Why there are no more heroes today like back then?" I didn't know that only a little later, my children would meet people like in those stories, people like diamonds: on whatever face you turned them, they were the same—honest, open, authentic, and true.

"Lord, have mercy, and give health to Joy." That is how

my children prayed for that angelic woman we met on the mountain.

She had a name of course, but that was what we nicknamed her, and that was how we prayed for her. I was amazed to find out that she lived no more than three kilometers away from us. It was like having a treasure and not knowing it had been near us. No day passed without receiving a phone call from her: "Have you found joy in the day? Be careful—I'll come over there with a stick if you haven't!"

It made me feel so alive and childish.

She had a troubling innocence, as if she had lived her whole life covered in a halo of joy and light.

I remember the first time she invited me to her home. I was breathless. All the walls of her large and spacious living room were covered with books and icons.

"Mom, Mom, it's like entering the famous library of Alexandria," Anthony said, fascinated by so many books.

Joy sat on the couch, thin and tall, with the face of a naughty and clever child, with her eyebrows slightly furrowed. She told me the life story of a saint, while holding my hands in her hands, delicate and strong at the same time. I remember how she told me, with the most gentle voice in the world: "See, Mioara, how much he suffered ... and how much confidence and love for Christ ..."

I sat down on the carpet at her feet and looked mortified. "When did she have time to read all those books?" I wondered. "And where did she get so much love and force of joy?"

I think she weighed no more than forty-five kilos, but I think her heart weighed as much as all the mountains in the

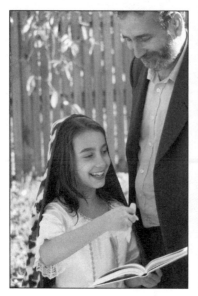
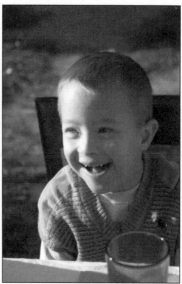

On this and the following page: Birthday party of Maria and Anthony at the home of the Grigore family, October 31, 2010. Photos by Florin Ivănescu. *Above left:* Maria and Viorel. *Above right:* Nektarios.

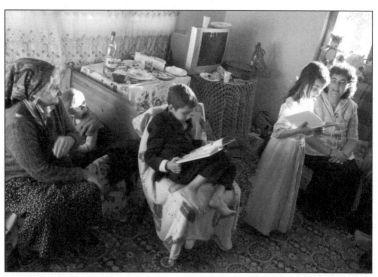

Left to right: Mioara's mother, Nektarios, Anthony, Maria, and Mioara.

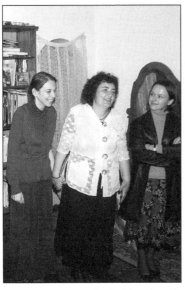

Mioara with friends (holding hands with "Joy").

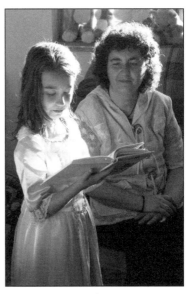

Maria and Mioara.

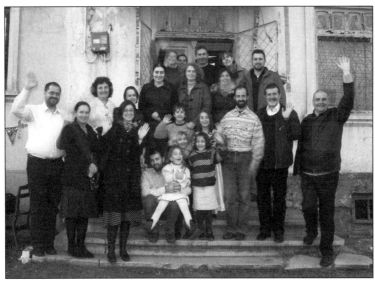

The Grigore family with friends.

world, or maybe even more. There were other times when she became so earthly. She was an expert in making bread. She made bread with olives, mushrooms, garlic, greens. When she invited me to lunch and gave me steaming bread, it was as if it were the first bread ever made on earth. Everything around her had the taste of beginning, clean and unaltered. One day, she started to dig ... and dug an entire garden alone. I could only imagine her with her back slightly arched, pushing the spade strongly into the ground, with her head toward the sky, thinking about saints, and with her feet firmly stuck into the ground.

To me, it was a huge contrast between heaven and earth, and a wonderful harmony between joy and suffering.

She was so simple, and she smelled so nice when she embraced me; she smelled like a mother and like incense. "Come to our church," she once told me before we parted.

And the next Sunday we did. It was a small church in the courtyard of a hospital. After the sermon, I looked carefully at the Father. He was as thin and tall as "Joy."

"My love," I informed my husband worriedly, "they're all thin in here. We're the only ones like pigs."

Indeed, since chemotherapy I had gained about ten kilos, which, in addition to the fifteen collected from five pregnancies, put me at more than seventy-five kilos. My husband was about eighty kilos.[1] We were ashamed to be seen like this....

---

[1] About one hundred sixty-five and one hundred seventy-six pounds, respectively.

MEETING SUPREME JOY

"Mommy, Mommy, the Father here looks like Don Quixote de La Mancha!" Maria told me in a loud voice.

"Maria, stop it!" I told her, explaining to her that we were not in a story or in a novel.

At first, both Viorel and I were intimidated by the priest. We felt like intruders. We felt as if somehow we disturbed the order and harmony of that church. Some time had to pass before I understood that Father was waiting for us to come to him, to open our souls, having immense patience with us. He did not push anything: neither the situation itself nor our behavior.... He let everything come from us. When I heard him saying once in a sermon, "Brethren, let us fall in love again with one another," it was as if I woke up from a dream. I remember it was spring, and I felt I was floating in an ocean of love. After the sermon, we went to the churchyard. I watched those people. I remember that from the beginning, a lady caught my attention. She was thin and delicate, too. She seemed so young, although she had white hair. I think she seemed so young because she had a petite figure. I saw her every Sunday sharing some small pills that people were not allowed to touch, coming out of a tube by turning a lid. "She could only be a doctor," I thought to myself. She looked like Greta Garbo. My children and I called her "Egret." She was like a swan, a white and ethereal swan. A swan that would enter my life with her big white wings, struggling almost every day with that black and monstrous swan that threatened to take me away from my children.

Egret would later do me the honor of becoming my soul sister, a sister whom I had longed for all my life.... And so I realized that the greatest horror of my life, my cancer, the terrifying disease, had actually given me two exceptional beings: a "joy" and a "swan," two beings who would teach me how to live differently, and especially how to think differently.

If only I had listened to them in everything....

29

Egret and Her Wonderful Pills

"Take this and that," and she showed me some small and round pills. "These pills twice a day, and the others three times."

Lord! And what names they had! Extremely complicated. I was wondering how she could remember so many formulas and elaborate names. She read a lot. She did not take my money and got angry when I over-thanked her.

If "Joy" was unreal in her joy, "Egret" was unreal in her modesty. She would give you the impression that you were her peer, even superior to her. I remember that one day she invited us to lunch. I was fascinated, and so were my husband and especially my children, at what we saw. She introduced us to her husband, a former general in the General Inspectorate for Emergency Situations. They were both alike. Until then, I had imagined that a general had to be somewhat unapproachable, with a big belly, bald, and with a serious face. Instead, we found a slender, lively, and extremely approachable general.... Smiling, he offered us a warm hand and made us feel at home. I looked at him more closely. He looked like Paul Newman.

He talked about everything and anything with real talent, dismissing from the beginning any inferiority complex that we might have had in front of him. A few days later, he did something that overwhelmed us.... We were at home when, all of a sudden, we looked out the window and saw a slender man entering the gate with some bags in his hands. When we looked more closely out the window, we realized it was the general. A general who brought us food and clothes for the children. He had a power to give and sacrifice that I had never thought to see in a general. He visited us every two or three weeks. He would call us in the morning and would inform us formally that in an hour and thirty-five minutes he would be at our place. He was amazing ... we all checked our watches. That was exactly how long it took him, not a minute more or less. He taught us exactly what punctuality and a word of honor meant. Discipline, and again discipline.

After his call, I could see the children running, dusting, washing the windows and floorboards quickly, hoping the general would find the cleanliness pleasing. "It's good to be visited by a general from time to time," I used to say to myself, looking at my five little children, who were cleaning with an enthusiasm unusual for their years.

I remember how, last year, he invited my husband and me to a famous restaurant in Bucharest for my birthday. This honored us a lot. It made me feel young and healthy again. It was a magnificent evening. I forgot about my illness, about my imminent death, and about my heartbreaking longing to be with my children. It made us feel that everything would be okay. I have never told him how much that evening meant to me. He was a general who would turn my entire system of values upside down, a general who would make me understand the immense complexity of his personality, little by little.

30

The Big Questions of My Life

"When are you going to have that CT?" Egret asked me, looking me in the eyes harder than Agent 007.

More than a year and a half had passed, and I, as if in a state of unconsciousness, obstinately refused to have it. Apparently, the doctor cared more about my life and my little children than I did. I preferred to be tied to a pole and whipped day and night than to find out that the disease had recurred and cancer had flooded my body.

"You know, Mom," said my son Anthony one morning, blinking impatiently with his lashes, with a large package of *Science World* magazines under his arm, "a recent discovery says that cancer cells actually communicate with each other, and use this basic mechanism, like bacteria, to spread in the body."

This information caused me dizziness. I could imagine how those awful cells communicated top-secret strategies and tactics to annihilate me faster. I felt like an ant squashed by the sole of a giant elephant.

On the other hand, every Sunday, Egret, always gentle and calm, inevitably reminded me of the CT. I didn't know how to explain to her that to me the CT actually meant a death sentence, which I was trying to postpone.

One had better send me to the electric chair than to a CT. I preferred a quick death, even if extremely violent, to a slow and agonizing one.

"Look, my sister," I said to her with a forced smile. "Look, my blood tests came out well! Even the tumor markers are good. It can't be anything serious!"

"Nonsense.... Don't you understand that you urgently need a CT?"

But I continued to live day by day lying to myself, believing that nothing had happened, and that in fact the cancer had not come back.... And so, one day I decided to return to work.

And that was that.

31

The Return

AFTER nearly nine years of staying at home, I decided to apply for a teaching position. I entered an imposing office and found myself in front of a school inspector. I had known him for at least ten years, since I had first been appointed as a teacher. He was the same gentle, calm, and patient man.

"Sir, I am a qualified teacher, I have five children and I have cancer … and I want to return to teaching after a nine-year gap."

He looked at me, smiling.

"My dear lady, I for one don't believe that you have cancer, nor that you have five little children.… You look too good."

I smiled back at him, and the next day, early in the morning I returned with all my five children to his office. There were about thirty people waiting, all school principals.

I asked an elderly, imposing, and respectable man, if I could go in with my children.

"Why?" he asked me puzzled.

"You know, the inspector doesn't believe that I have given birth to five children in seven years without there being any twins."

"But the question is: are any of them his?" he asked, leaning his head slightly towards me and winking cheekily.

I smiled mechanically, slightly discouraged by the bad joke, and asked him again.

"Be my guest," the man replied cordially.

My children entered one by one into the office. The inspector's puzzlement was directly proportional to the number of children who walked through the door.

"You know, these are my children, and this is Anthony, if you want to ask him questions."

"What grade are you in, my child?"

"Fourth," replied Anthony.

"What should I ask you, my child? Tell me, what do you want to talk about? Have you heard of 'pi'?"

"You mean the famous 'pi,' which has 2.7 trillion decimal places?"

They then talked about the Doppler Effect, something about String Theory, and then about the Small World Theory.

Beads of sweat covered his forehead. After a while he took my boy into his arms and with tears in his eyes told him in a choked voice, "You will find a cure for cancer, you hear me? You should become a famous doctor." And he embraced him and the other children.

The air in the office was heavy with emotion. We parted with the promise that we would meet again soon and we hurried home.

On the way back, Anthony begged me, "Mommy, Mommy, please let me sit in front, I'll wear my seat belt. Please, just for five minutes."

For his sake and without much thought, I let him sit in front and I went to the back seat with the other kids. It didn't take longer than three minutes for a police officer to stop us.

"What's with the kid in front?" he asked, and then requested to see my husband's license.

I watched from the back seat with my heart racing. He was tall, solid, sober and especially full of himself. He was aware of all his power of action and decision.

Suddenly, I saw Anthony jumping from his seat, out of the car, in front of the police officer, and told him in a very excited voice, "Mr. Policeman, please, don't fine my daddy! You know, I was born with a genetic condition and that's why I'm so tall, but actually I'm six months old, and I have a disabled brother, and my mother is also disabled...."

Mortified at what I heard, I watched how the poor police officer made his eyes as huge as onions, came closer, and looked inside the car at us.

I immediately smiled, with a stupid face. Nektarios laughed at the police officer, and Maria, Macrina, and Justina waived at him, laughing.

Suddenly, I saw an expression of sympathy, tolerance, and overwhelming compassion on the face of the police officer.

He was becoming increasingly aware that he had found a car full of disabled people, and in a trembling and rushed voice, he told us to leave urgently, handing my husband's documents back, without any fine. We all shook our heads, humble and docile, thanking him more than was needed, and we drove away.

On the way home, I scolded my child that he had lied with

such ease to a police officer. He cried remorsefully, tears flooding his cheeks while he was looking out the window. I knew he was a very sensitive child, who would cry at anything, but I did not expect him to cry so badly. He sighed and cried all the way home.

I remembered him crying that badly only twice before. Once, when we were out of money and food, and I asked them all to pray to St. Nicholas. And because he was crying while praying, I thought that Anthony was probably impressed by the life of St. Nicholas, but I was wrong. Later he told me that I should never ask him to pray to a saint for money or food because he felt ashamed. The other time was when we were coming home from the hospital after a chemo session. It was freezing outside. We were all in the car going home. I asked Viorel to stop the car so I could throw up.

As I started to throw up I turned my head away, and I saw two prostitutes scantily dressed and with a lot of makeup on the side of the road.

I remember that while throwing up, the entire planet moved with me, and I had a moment of revolt and told my husband, "Look at them, they don't get cancer …"

Then I realized that all the kids had heard me. I looked first at Anthony, terrified of what a stupid thing I had said, and he, with tears rushing down both cheeks, begged his father, "Dad, Daddy, tell those girls to come to our house so we can dress them and cover them, so they won't catch a cold, Daddy …"

He felt so much pity for them, and cried!

After him, a few seconds later, Justina started to cry, too, and then Nektarios, and in the end Macrina and Maria.

We were in a car full of children who cried for those "loose women," whom the kids saw only as poor naked and frozen girls. I realized then with horror the enormous distance between my frozen heart and the innocence of my children. I realized with sadness that the cancer would not go away from me in any way as long as I did not fight for a radical change in my way of thinking and especially of feeling.

Indeed, I have never felt more stupid than on that day.

The cold penetrated deep into my bones.

All the way home I could no longer say a word. At night, among unrelated sporadic dreams and nightmares with car accidents and falls into voids, I dreamed I was sitting on the side of the highway, wearing skimpy clothes and vulgar makeup, stopping truck drivers and negotiating with them. I was one of those women. It was tragic and curious that I was not bothered by the situation. A truck with a sign saying "Viorel" on the windshield stopped. It was him, the driver of my life. When I woke up, all sweaty, I realized the situation: What if I was the true harlot? And for the first time, that morning I realized that something could be even more frightening than cancer … my soul, my soul bound and strangled with such fiery chains. "Where will my soul go, my God?" I wondered, terrified. I did not expect an answer.… I was so tired and lonely … and the highway from my dream was waiting for me, the highway on which my soul roamed.… I was so tired …

32

Aida and Her Notary Documents

"This is Aida." Egret introduced me to a thin, delicate, and ethereal lady, on a Sunday after the church service. She was a notary. Her angelic body was in striking contrast to her job. How could so many laws, paragraphs, legal definitions, and especially all kinds of notary documents fit inside of her? She wore glasses and seemed very intellectual. I didn't know how to stand around her. I felt uncultured. She smiled to me and handed me a delicate but strong hand at the same time.

Later I would realize what inner strength this lady had. She possessed a huge power of sacrifice for her neighbor. I did not expect my life to be prolonged by a handful of people. Sometimes, I was embarrassed to leave my home to go to that miraculous place, which was the little church in the hospital courtyard, because all those wonderful people who sacrificed for me were physically thin, delicate, and extremely sensitive. I, despite being poisoned and irradiated, had a weight so visible and considerable that I would have hidden myself in the nearest cave or burrow.

And that was nothing: I had an appetite so big that if I had seen a pig running down the street I would have been able to bite into it, if common sense didn't stop me.

I had an inferiority complex. Joy, Egret, Aida, and the other heroes of my children bought me monthly herbal remedies of high value (both financial and medical). I needed a strong immune system. However, they strengthened my soul even more than my body. I never thought that so much love could be possible between people, I never thought that so much sacrifice could exist, especially for me, a stranger.

"This is my husband," Aida introduced me on a Sunday to a tall man with green eyes and an athletic stature, resembling a Russian character from one of Nikita Mikhalkov's movies.[1]

He was an engineer but he seemed to be the quintessence of all engineers on the planet.

Being an expert on the subject, he brought the great inventor Nikola Tesla into our lives.[2] He told us so many stories about him that the little ones really fell in love with this great inventor. I could hear them praying for him every night.

"Lord, save Mr. Tesla's soul!"

"Mommy, Mommy," Anthony would say every night, "Do you know this amazing man developed the alternating current, the radio, wireless transmission techniques, the remote control, the electric vehicle concept, and especially electrotherapy?"

The engineer told me that, according to these therapies,

---

[1] Mikhalkov (1945–) is one of Russia's most acclaimed film directors.

[2] Tesla (1856–1943) was a Serbian-American electrical engineer, mechanical engineer, and physicist, whose contributions have had a tremendous impact on modern technology. There has been a resurgence of public interest in him since the 1990s.

if the human body was penetrated by electric currents and vibrations, tissues could heal.

The truth is that for nearly three years I had taken all kinds of pills, of all sizes and colors. I had drunk all kinds of liquids, which I then threw up. On top of that, a lady told me about some wonder pills that had healed her dying kitten, and another lady told me how she had healed her paralyzed dog with some fish pills.

Dogs and cats miraculously cured, powder made of beetles, mushrooms from places still unspoiled, enzymatic liquids, you name it, I had tried them all. But having electricity passing through me, at who knows what voltage, indeed, that I had not experienced.

And yet, I remember, on an autumn morning, I woke up determined to clean the kitchen. I started by painting the walls. I used to love the smell of fresh primer—it reminded me of the clean smell of my grandparents' house, with the floors clean and sheets freshly washed. I remember how, when I was little, my grandmother took me on a country road, where we gathered horse manure; at home we mixed it with earth and straw, and with it we repaired the floor. Even now, after decades, there are times when I recall that smell of fresh manure and painted walls like a beautiful dream. Everything was so simple and clean.

But let's return to one of the greatest inventors of all time, whom the engineer had brought into our lives. Speaking of electro-therapy, that morning I started to paint the walls. My husband was not at home, and the children were at school or kindergarten. I wanted to surprise them. At some point,

I reached a half-exposed wall socket, which my husband had postponed fixing. With a brush wet with primer in hand, I cheerfully painted. I remember that I was thinking about Nikola Tesla. Light-headed, as usual, I reached with the brush directly into the socket wires.... And then it started, and it went on and on. It was like falling into the latrine of my childhood.... The shaking began, the jerking began, and I could not stop. I strained myself so hard, as if I could have broken into a million pieces. I felt like I was made of glass and someone was breaking me with a huge sledgehammer.... I kept shaking, and I could not think of anything except that I would crumble, and billions of particles from me would stick to the walls like that white primer. I felt that the ordeal would not last long. It didn't resemble any pain I had experienced before. It was like an implosion. I felt I could no longer stand, and for a split second, I stopped fighting ... just like when I was seven and covered by that mountain of sewage. I only wanted to sleep, to disappear, to pass into nothingness. And then, for a split second, I saw the image of my five little children crying over losing me. With a huge effort, I managed to release the brush and I was freed. I fell next to the bed, powerless. It was as if I had fought in all the wars of the earth.

After a few minutes, I felt somewhat relieved: "So, I tried your electro-therapy after all, Mr. Tesla!" Maybe I had electrocuted those cursed cancer cells.

That day, I felt hope taking shape in my heart. The hope that I might live, that the cancer might leave me like that electric current. I loved Tesla enormously at that moment, and I especially loved those people who had arrived in my life like angels, with huge wings and seraphic smiles. I enormously loved Egret with her general. I loved Joy with her three little children. I loved the notary with her engineer.

What intrigued me and made me admire the engineer enormously, was his respect and love for his parents. They had both gone to God. In their names, he performed charity. He thought of them all the time. When we went to monasteries and wrote their names on prayer lists, I would get tears in my eyes when I thought about how much he continued to love his parents. A love beyond death. I wished enormously that at least one of my five children would pray for me as much when I was gone.

Blessed parents, privileged parents, for having such a son.

33

The Plumber and His "Living" Word

"WHEN are you going to do that CT?" Egret asked me again, tired and weary of my cowardice. I could not make any more excuses, and I felt I might slowly lose her friendship. That would have devastated me completely. I did not know what to do anymore. I was stuck because of my own weakness, a weakness that had created such a fake world for me. Like I had been shoved into a huge CT scanner for years and could not get out of it. A CT scanner that was ticking like my heart and every tick was a lost day; I was losing more and more days and I could not get out of it.... I would wake up in the morning all sweaty, and was no longer able to tell the difference between what was real and what was not in my life.

I felt this way until one morning, when a man from Joy's church came to our house. He was as tall and thin as everyone else, a little bald and bearded. He looked amazingly like St. Nicholas.

He was a plumber, and he had come to install running water and a sink in the kitchen. It was a dream come true to have running water in the kitchen. I watched him take out, from a large bag, dozens of screws, wrenches, and nuts, each with its specific role. At every screw and nut he tightened, he uttered, "Glory to Thee, O Lord!" He tightened, added a faucet, and a "Glory be to God for all things!"

I watched him, perplexed, as he worked for six hours that day and had already told us half of the *Paterikon*. I saw how he applied Orthodoxy to screws, nuts, and faucets. I felt thousands of light years away from him.

He lived and worked only for Christ. How could such a person exist? "And a plumber," I thought, completely puzzled. But that was nothing. I remember one day when he told us how someone hit his car in the parking lot. He had an old Volvo, about twenty years old. He needed it in order to feed his family. It was hit pretty badly. Then, our plumber got out of the car and with a gentleness worthy of St. Nicholas said to the driver responsible for the accident, "It's all right, Brother. This happened because of my sins. Forgive me, a sinner."

The man looked at him speechless. I think he was more shocked by these words than by the accident itself. He didn't know what to do. The humility of the plumber completely perplexed him. He could not recover. I don't know the ending, but the fact is that wherever he went, he turned things upside down, and changed ways of thinking, feeling, and even loving.

He refocused the human mind; he took it up somewhere into a world without sin or passion.

I looked at him and I could not believe it. It was as if a breach in time would appear in our house when he entered: a piece of the timeless Egyptian and Romanian *Paterikons* came into my kitchen—simplicity in its purest form. I had been given yet another hero. He would tell me, "You're in the front line. Let's fight together."

He gave me strength. He had three children and a fourth coming soon. He worked up to fourteen hours a day. He was in demand by many people.

"How much will this cost me?" he would be asked after working for weeks.

"As much as you want," the plumber would reply. He would be given a symbolic sum, or even nothing.

"Thank you, thank you."

He would shake hands warmly with the man for whom he had worked, and he would go home tired, penniless, but with the great satisfaction that he had made someone happy.

His wife would wait patiently on their porch. She was docile and understanding, even when her husband came home without money for the thousandth time.

But it didn't matter. In their home, peace and harmony reigned, and most of all, love ruled.

34

Plescoi Sausages

"Hold your breath," the hoarse voice of the doctor rang relentlessly in my ears.

"Tick, tick, tick," responded the CT scanner. Its sound reminded me of a deadly curse: the cancer cells had not died, and they romped like crazy throughout my body, invading it.

I felt like I would be in that CT scanner for an eternity. While I was inside, the air became increasingly insufficient. It was as if I had made a breach in time and I was in the latrine of my childhood, where I could barely breathe. The only difference was that the latrine had not ticked like the CT scanner, and had never told me that five little children would remain without a mother.

"Hold your breath," the doctor told me with a hoarse voice. I obeyed and I did not breathe. He left the office and I was still holding my breath; my heart was ready to implode in my chest. When I felt that I could no longer resist, I started to breathe slowly, slowly, obviously feeling very guilty, like I had put a bomb in that CT scanner. I was breathing almost imperceptibly. When I heard the door opening again, after about ten minutes, I began to hold my breath again, as conscientious as a diligent student.

"Haven't you breathed until now?" The doctor asked me, slightly puzzled. "Well, that's fine; continue to hold your breath!"

I did not know why he focused so much on my lungs. "I am sure he will find cancer in my liver," I thought. It didn't cross my mind that the malignant cells might have made their nest in my lungs. Many thousands of cells, or whatever the doctor wrote on that white, immaculate sheet of paper. The big black writing seemed alive and undulated on the sheet, wavy and tragic at the same time, like a highly poisonous snake. It described my lungs with a rigor worthy of the *Guinness Book of World Records*. I was so rich. I had everything in my lungs: three inches of water, interstitial metastases, lymph nodes, two lumps, etc. It was a labyrinth in there. Only the Minotaur was missing. Or maybe even he was there. I had a sick, obsessive, pathological fear of these metastases. Suddenly, I became calm. I had finally gotten out of my own hell, the hell of my helplessness. Why had I struggled for two years with the worst thoughts, but hadn't tried to free myself?

I was so happy to be free. It didn't matter that my lungs were actually "melting" into water; I was glad that I had gotten rid of doubt, fear, and the black wings of death that strangled me little by little like Poe's raven.

"Okay, my love, let's go!"

I took my husband's hand and we left the hospital. Outside, I inhaled once strongly, as if that breath would have been enough to live my whole life on. Neither Viorel nor I said anything on the way home. I watched him closely. His face had an intense gray color, his eyes were very troubled, and his hands were strained on the steering wheel, as if a bomb were inevitably going to detonate. I wanted to burst into tears, but I could not.... I thought about those two years in which I had obstinately refused to get a CT scan, I thought about how I had hoped with an insane intensity. Terrified and frightened, I admitted for the first time the supremacy and especially the victory of the cancer cells. They had defeated me. For the past two years, I had swallowed all kinds of tinctures, teas, and pills of all types and colors: red, white, green, blue, purple. I had swallowed all living colors. Everyone had urged me, advised me and begged me not to eat anything that could feed the cancer cells. Although I had gained over ten kilos, I had stopped eating meat, sugar, and dairy products. I thought that this way I would starve the cursed cancer cells. But those cells were not dying, not disappearing, not even sleeping. They had multiplied with an astonishing vitality. They had the intelligence of thousands of years of survival. Anthony once read to me that even Tutankhamun had prostate cancer. Tutankhamun and I—two people defeated in the battle with these super cells. I could imagine them: black, hairy, with huge tentacles, vibrant, active, and intelligent, using a cunning attack strategy.

I could not understand. I had felt no pain in my lungs for two years, I was not getting tired and, in addition, I had had many X-rays. All for nothing. The cancer had devastated my lungs. Insidiously, easily, steadily, with millimeter precision, and barely perceptibly, the metastases were conquering me each day. "The cancer cell has not died. Long live the cancer cell," I said to myself.

After two years of vain hopes, I said in a masterful tone

to my husband, "Take me to the nearest pub!" He did not ask why. We arrived in front of a deli that had four tables full of empty beer bottles. Inside, tired and bored workers were drinking and smoking. I watched them. They were dirty and smelled of bad drinks, tobacco, and sweat. They all swore and seemed to be healthy. "Don't they have lung metastases?" I wondered rhetorically, watching them smoking with unbelievable craving. With the look of a hungry animal, I checked the cabinet. There, in grandeur worthy of a royal house, lay thick salamis, ham cooked in cabbage sauce, smoked loin fillets, and smoked bacon. Instantly, my mouth began to water. I swallowed quickly and panted as if I had suddenly gone into labor, my eyes remaining fixed on some sausages: the famous Plescoi sausages that I always loved. I wanted something strong, something so strong it would burn. I wanted a taste so peppery, salty, and spicy that it would bring tears to my eyes. I wanted to cry from the sausages and not from cancer.

"All the sausages in the cabinet, please," I ordered like a rich gypsy king.

I looked at them avidly as they were weighed. Thin, thick, traditional, full of meat, onion, garlic, pepper: sausages waiting to be taken, to be mine forever. I also got two liters of beer, paid hastily, and went to the car. My husband was staring at the sausages, but he dared not ask me anything.

When we arrived home, I did not even undress. I quickly took a pan from the cupboard, put it on the stove, threw in some fat from last year's pig, and began to fry the sausages. It was a night with a full moon. Suddenly, the courtyard filled with the smell of sausages. I sniffed the smell like a predator. I loved it. I savored it. It made me feel so alive! Viorel was in a corner of the kitchen, kind of stunned. He sat at a small table and he looked so gray. He was as motionless as a rock. Time froze in our kitchen, and all that could be sensed was the smell of sausages. The kids were sleeping peacefully in their room. I could hear on the radio, in the background, a traditional song from Oltenia. I quickly prepared some polenta. Its intense yellow color fit perfectly with the music. I was red, sweaty, and especially desperate. I felt the urge for revenge. To avenge my two years of cowardice, my despair and anxieties, to avenge myself on those sneaky cells. That night with a full moon — the most wonderful moon I had ever seen — it seemed like those sausages fried in lard, with their vivid, sharp and primitive scent, would be the answer to my entire existential tragedy. It was as if time had expanded. I mixed the polenta, and its hot steam seemed to come from my brain and not from the pot. I had been waiting for this for so long. It seemed almost like a historic moment.

For more than seven hundred days, I had wanted to eat these sausages. I remember that one Christmas, Egret's general brought us home two kilos[1] of these sausages. After preparing them, I called my husband and children to eat, and I went to another room so as not to faint from craving. I remember that all that night I dreamed of climbing Mount Everest. I wore an oxygen mask and a huge backpack. And I climbed and climbed and it was more and more difficult. When we reached the top, full of ecstasy and joy, I realized

---

[1] About four and a half pounds.

that the mountain was not a normal mountain—it was a mountain of sausages. I had reached the top of a mountain of sausages.

Now, my time had come. I took some polenta and put it next to the sausages. The taste was good! I closed my eyes for a minute, and I felt like I was floating. I felt an immense happiness. Fat dribbled down my fingers, so I licked them. I did not want to lose any drop of fat. At that moment, the most precious diamond did not equal the smallest drop of fat. I did not want to lose anything. I ate a sausage, two, three. I ate enough for a lifetime. I was greasy. I had fat on my fingers, cheeks, even in my brain. I savored it and I felt like I was floating in an ocean of fat.

I quickly filled a large glass of the worst quality beer and drank it. Viorel was in a state of total shock. He looked at me, appalled and resigned at the same time. He felt that he had lost me forever. After I wolfed the sausages and polenta and drank the beer down with incredible speed, the inevitable occurred: I burped with a noise hard to describe, scattering sausage smells into the air, smells that reminded me that I was the woman of my husband, the woman of my man, of the peasant beside whom I wanted to grow old....

Later, we went outside on the porch. I lifted my eyes to the sky. Thousands of stars participated in our silence. I did not have anything to say to my husband or to my children. I felt like a failure. At one point under the moonlight and stars, Viorel Grigore, my husband, took me by the hand and, looking into my eyes, said with a trembling voice, "Please, I beg you, don't give up the fight." I could not reply. I would have given anything not to disappoint him, but I had already given up.

Spy cells, cancer cells, had invaded me. They were a part of me; they were ten, a thousand, a million times smarter than me. They annihilated me completely. Only one spot was left to conquer, my heart. In it there were so many wonderful beings that I loved desperately, stubbornly, painfully. My man was holding my arm ... and I was so sad.... All my life I had wanted and sought to be brave. I kept saying to myself, "If I could live up to the moment ..." I wanted to live with dignity, worthily and courageously, and I had educated my children to do the same. And what was I? I was fat, terrified of death, excited by the smell of sausages and poor beer, and I burped like a truck driver who was tired and tipsy after a day of work. That night, we sat on the porch. My husband and I watched the sky studded with stars and listened to the crickets' song. The feeling of defeat was awful.

"But what if I had lost the battle and not the entire war? What if the next day I would start all over and return to the front lines? What if God gave me a little more time? Maybe now I would know what to do with this time."

However, whatever I did, I would probably still remain a deserter.

And so, tired and resigned, I fell asleep with my head on my husband's shoulder.... It had been a year since my dream, and that night I had a similar one.... I was climbing Mount Everest again, only this time it was not a mountain of sausages. I was at its base and started to try to climb it. This time it was a mountain of metastases. It was the mountain of my death. I heard the voices of my children from the other side of the mountain. I needed to climb it, to get to my angels ... and so, I started to climb.... And I returned to the front lines, to the front lines of my heart.

35

Nights with Stories and Water in My Lungs

I RETURNED to the hospital. I felt remorseful and I had chills. Chills of cowardice and especially shame. I felt a terrible shame in front of the doctor.... She had fought desperately for my life. For two years, I hadn't even come back once to thank her. I felt like one of the nine lepers.[1]

"Will you take me back?" I asked, avoiding her eyes. She smiled at me. That smile was worth a thousand words. It encouraged me a lot.

I started the chemo again. My breathing became increasingly more difficult. My life had now, as in the beginning, a taste of poison. The tumor markers had reached eight hundred. My children were going to school. Macrina became more mature every day. At school, she took care of Justina and Nektarios. She came home sad. "Why do children call my brother stupid?" she asked with tears in her eyes. I tried to tell her that Nektarios's condition could not be understood by other children. Justina's teacher was exasperated by her. She could not

---

[1] A reference to the Gospel account in which Christ healed ten lepers, but only one returned to thank Him (Luke 17:11–19).

understand addition and subtraction. However, she was great with words. She easily played with them. I remember how one day Justina entered the house like a storm, coming home from school tired and nervous, and told me, "Leave me, leave me alone. I'm tired. I have to love my country … that's what my teacher told us. And what should I do to love it faster?"

I looked at her bemused. For a long time, I had not thought whether I really love my country. Where was my patriotic feeling? Was I a complete brute?

I carried on with the chemo for three weeks. The markers did not want to drop at all. Justina continued not to understand mathematics. "Mom, why should I put the numbers one below the other? Why not next to each other?" One day, coming from preschool, tired as usual, she asked me thoughtfully, "Mommy, can lice also get lice on their heads? Today we were checked for lice."

I do not know what I answered; the fact was that out of twenty-one days, at least seventeen days I was not able to do anything. Nausea reigned again in my body more forcefully and violently than ever.

I remember that once, after coming home from school, Maria, my oldest daughter, gathered all her siblings in a corner of the room and told them, "Don't tell Mommy that you're hungry. Otherwise, I'll get mad at you if you don't listen to me. None of you are hungry, you understand?"

"But …," Justina tried to reply.

"Okay, I said something, and you have to listen to me, because I'm the eldest.…"

She did not know I was in the next room. She did not

know that her words, full of love and compassion, hurt me enormously.

Only then did I realize that, in fact, Maria was being my mother and I was the daughter. My sickness had added a hundred years to her. I had stolen her childhood. I had stolen her playfulness, her carefree attitude, the spring of innocent thoughts. I had given her a cold and frosty winter of hundreds of years. That hurt me the most. She had just started the fifth grade, but she acted as if she had already graduated high school.

I remember that one afternoon, being out of bread, I went downstairs with her to the kitchen to mix some flour and water and knead some dough. We did not have enough flour, and I felt as if I did not have enough air either, but instead I had the force of my daughter's heart.

"Dear," she said with gravity in her voice, "you lie there on the bed, and I'll knead."

I looked at her, at how she touched the flour with her thin and long little fingers, with enormous care not to waste anything. Macrina came downstairs, too, shy and withdrawn as usual, and murmured in a low voice, "Can I help, Mommy?"

"Listen, dear," Maria immediately replied, "go upstairs— we're already two women here!"

I could not believe it. I watched her bent over the bowl of flour, how she carefully kneaded the dough. She had flour on her nose and cheek, and she kneaded the bread with so much love, and with such a pure soul.

"Please, smile for me, Mom! You're tense again."

But I didn't know how I felt. I did not know whom I was

looking at kneading the bread: my daughter or my mother. I quickly went outside. I went to the garden to cry. When I returned to the house trying to smile, Maria told me in a slightly raised voice, "Hey, dear, if you want to accept the inevitable, that's your problem. I know what I say to Lord-Lord[2] every night."

I remained silent with guilt. During this period of my awful and unequal battle with cancer, I had never asked God to heal me. As long as I did not believe it was possible, I could not ask for something like this.... I had asked only to be allowed to see my little children, even poisoned as I was, to be among them for a little longer. The illness itself did not hurt the most, but the helplessness that it generated.

I could not cook, I could not do laundry, and, most of all, I could not tell stories to them. I longed for the evenings and nights when I had read them stories. They had to work a lot: they were cleaning, cooking, and caring for two sick women. My eighty-year-old mother had fallen sick and was in bed. Maria and Macrina were, in fact, caring for two dying people.

As soon as I came home from chemo I would scream, "Maria, quickly get me a bucket!" My mother from her room was also crying, "Maria, I need the bedpan." Once, Maria, running between me and her grandmother, raised her eyes and with her face beaming with joy told me, "Mommy, Mommy, I know what I'll do when I grow up: I'll get a job at a nursing

---

[2] The Romanian expression "Lord-Lord" (*Doamne-Doamne*) is often used when teaching children how to pray, and thus by children in their prayers.

home. I feel I've found my vocation." I watched her carrying the bedpan, the bucket, the burden of two sick people.

Meanwhile, on the side where my breast had been removed, my hand had swollen a lot. Twenty lumps had been removed, but the lymph was not draining properly. "You have elephantiasis," the doctor told me very seriously. My hand became more and more swollen and more hideous. It really looked like an elephant's trunk.

"Keep your hand up all the time; it's the only solution," the doctors told me unanimously. But I didn't listen to them. I had so many things to do. Also, my nails became blue and started to fall off from the chemo. I had brown, black, blue nails—all colors. But that was not the problem; the big problem was the awful smell. My nails smelled like dead flesh, as if I were rotting alive. I was so embarrassed when my husband and children hugged me. I hid my hands behind my back, but I was still stinking. I used a lot of creams, soaps, and perfumes, but it was all in vain. The stench of death, of sin, of dissolution poured out of me with incredible power.

"Mom, Mom," Justina called me one evening, "I'm scared!"

"Why, my baby?" I asked her, full of worry.

"Who does all these bad things to you? Who beats you over your nails so that they're so black and smell so bad?"

The only thing I could tell her was that Mommy was happy to be with all five of them no matter what. I watched her frown, and her dimples deepened even more. She was thinking very hard and tried to find answers to all her questions.

"Mommy, if you have only one hand and one breast, do you only have half a brain?"

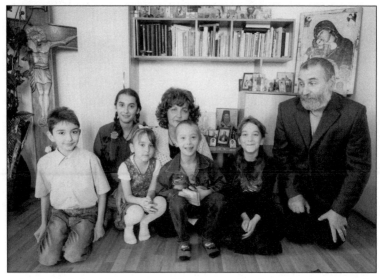

On this and the following page: The Grigore family at their home, April 9, 2014. Photos by the well-known Romanian photographer Dinu Lazăr. *Above, left to right:* Anthony, Maria, Justina, Mioara, Nektarios, Macrina, and Viorel.

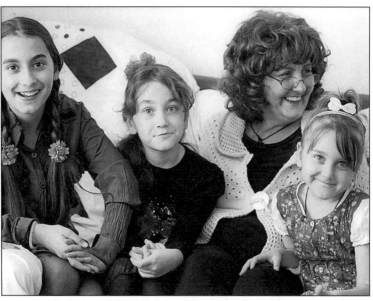

Left to right: Maria, Macrina, Mioara, and Justina.

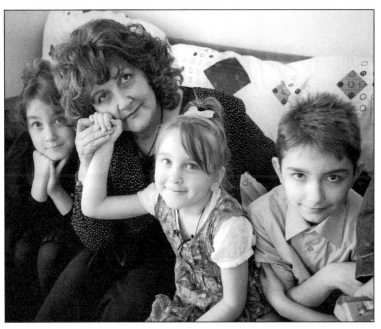

Left to right: Macrina, Mioara, Justina, and Anthony.

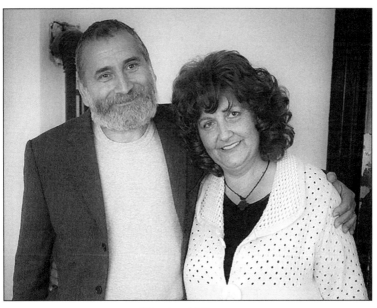

Viorel and Mioara.

And although I was going to the most hidden corner of my house, all my five little children would find me and start to soothe me. Macrina caressed my back, Nektarios put his hands on my forehead, Maria brought me a basin with hot water, Anthony read me a list of herbal remedies, and Justina made up stories to entertain me. And so began the magic of stories invented by my youngest daughter.

"Mom, this is a short story—can I tell it to you?"

I nodded through attacks of convulsive coughing.

"Once upon a time, there was an apple that had eyes, a nose, and a mouth, and this apple started on a journey, on a long path, where he met a man, and that man bit him once, but then, looking into the apple's eyes, he felt so sorry for what he did, so sorry, that they lived happily ever after."

And then I would stop coughing. I would forget about everything, forget even to cough, while I was listening to the stories of my five-year-old girl. I would forget about the water in my lungs and let myself be transported into the overwhelmingly innocent world of the apple with eyes and mouth, and especially of the little bee—the little bee that made a major and drastic decision concerning her life. "Once upon a time, there was a lonely bee that flew from flower to flower. A man saw her one day and gave her a flower. The bee was very impressed with the gesture, and she started to think, and kept asking herself, 'Why did I want to sting him?' And she decided to cut her stinger off. And so, they lived happily ever after."

In those moments nothing mattered anymore. She was so sweet and soft. I held her as I looked out the window at the stars and moon pouring pale light into our bedroom.

I remained speechless. What if God had spoken through her?

"You have to do a CT scan on your brain, because cancer goes from the lungs to the brain eventually."

"I will, Doctor," I reassured her, because there had been nights when I lost my vision, fractions of time when I could not see at all, so in any case I had to do a CT scan on my brain.

"My sister," I asked Egret one day, "if I have cancer in my brain, does that mean I'll no longer be able to think?"

I was terrified at the prospect.

"My dear," Egret responded calmly, "you haven't been thinking much anyway since you got married."

I loved her so much then. She had an overflowing sense of humor, sometimes dry, typically English, but it felt so good.

"Do you think that I have any chance to live for another three, six months?"

I clung desperately to her answer.

"I don't know how many months you have, but you have at least six hours...."

She had a way that gave me wings.

The fact was that Justina's question as to whether I had half a brain determined me to quickly get a CT scan of my brain, too. I was going through the most difficult, the most awful period of my life. The cough would not let me breathe. It was a delirious cough, which dominated my nights. At night, the cough manifested itself freely. The water in my lungs rose, and I started to cough. I coughed with incredible violence, as if an infinite number of hearts were exploding within me.

Sometimes, I screamed at my children to go away from me. I was afraid that I would contaminate them with death and decay, but they did not listen at all. They suffocated me with their love. Every evening they warmed up a sock with salt in it, and that sock with salt was passed from hand to hand until finally it arrived on my back. Every night they covered me with salt and with their hands.

Night after night, the only noise in the house was my heavy, loud cough. I coughed with such violence. One night, ten nights, twenty nights — all nights seemed so long and endless. Nights spent in complete helplessness and lack of air. I remember that on one of those nights, unable to endure it any longer, I clung desperately to my husband's neck and implored him, "I beg you, take me to the hospital to remove the water from my lungs! I can't bear it anymore — don't you understand?"

"Even if I saw you fainting in front of me, I still wouldn't take you there, my love! You only need a little bit of patience. It's better this way."

He shook my shoulders, hugged me to his chest, and covered me with hot salt. "Okay, okay, my love, it will pass." He was so strong and sure of himself. Eight centimeters of water had accumulated in my lungs, but his love for me was like an infinity of centimeters. It was good to listen to him. If he didn't want to allow all kinds of needles into my lungs, I had to trust his intuition. I knew I had to have patience, but the only problem was I had neither patience nor air. This continuous cough and lack of air tired me a lot.

"Mommy, Mommy, let me tell you another story. Once

upon a time, there was a dusty and dirty light bulb, but he felt happy the way he was. He did not know how it felt to be lit, because all his life he had been dusty and unlit. Until one night, a boy entered the room and lit the light bulb. And, Mommy, the bulb was so scared that he exploded. He broke into pieces, Mommy, because he did not know what it was like to shine, and he broke from so much happiness."

I probably would have exploded as well, if by some miracle I had been healed and could stay among my children.

And so, night after night, on those long, endless, and frosty winter nights, the miracle of Justina's stories kept me alive.

And how they prayed! I heard them from the next room, praying with my cough in the background. I liked how Anthony, when he prayed, didn't have the courage to ask for too much. "God, if You will, please, remove at least 1.5 to 1.7 centimeters out of the 8 centimeters of water." He was so delicate in his prayers.

Justina prayed all the time with a doll in her arms, an old doll that had a hole in her back. I could hear her: "God, my doll has water in her lungs. See the hole in her back? Please heal them both." She was so convincing.

They kept me alive with their pure and innocent prayers—prayers of vulnerable, scared, compassionate children, who had aged too soon.

The water was absorbed from my lungs by the little hands of Nektarios caressing my bald head, by the bags with warm salt placed by Maria on my chest, by the information read by Anthony from his encyclopedias, by the foot massage given to

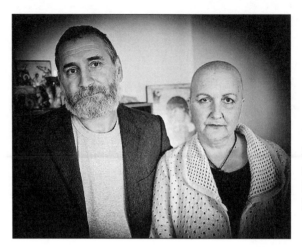

Viorel and Mioara, April 9, 2014.
Photo by Dinu Lazăr.

me by Macrina, by the stories of Justina, and especially by the stubbornness of my husband to fight to the last drop of blood for my life, his obstinacy not to let anything separate us. Not even death.

36
Suleiman the Magnificent of Romania

I WAS always accompanied by a shiver. The feeling of being cold practically became one with me. My feet, my hands, my heart, and all my organs were trembling in a crazy and agonizing dance, a never-ending dance. Then, like a last-minute rescue, I met a man who would have an overwhelming influence on me. He looked strikingly like "Suleiman the Magnificent," the character from the famous TV series with the same name.[1] He had a wonderful wife and five gorgeous daughters between five and fifteen years old. He often went to Mount Athos, with a power of sacrifice and dedication hard to describe in words. He was so indebted to banks that it would take him at least 1,050 years to pay it off. He said to me, "My little sister, the solution to my problems is no longer from this world." He went to the Holy Mountain and there he gave himself to prayer.

[1] Originally titled *Muhteşem Yüzyıl* (The Magnificent Century), this Turkish television series was based on the life of the longest-reigning sultan of the Ottoman Empire. It was very popular in Romania, where it was known as *Süleyman Magnificul*.

The pain in my right shoulder, hands, and feet became unbearable. One night, around 11 p.m., I received a call from the Magnificent: "I think I've found a solution. I think it'll work for you, too." With a glimmer of hope, thinking immediately of a miraculous treatment from Greece, I almost begged him to come and bring it to me even that night, since I was unable to endure the cruel and merciless pain in my bones.

He said to me, "Go to a room, face a wall, and draw a circle. Focus for a while on that circle and then start to bang your head against it. And do it until the pain in your head overshadows all other pain."

I remained speechless for a moment. Was he serious? I thanked him kindly, and I imagined myself on that frosty winter night banging my big and stupid head against the walls repeatedly, making the pain in my bones disappear as if by a miracle. I wished the pain would subside a bit so I could follow his crazy advice. I felt as if I hadn't slept for a thousand years. Around 4 a.m., I could not endure the pains any longer, so I snuck into the children's room, took a piece of chalk from a bag, and drew a circle large enough for my head.

At first, I approached the wall somewhat shyly, and I tapped my head inside the circle lightly, slowly, with fear and caution. The result was far from satisfactory.... It did not hurt enough. I was disgusted with my own cowardice, so I went to the opposite corner of the room, determined to finally do something decisive in my life. I rushed toward the wall and hit my head in the right spot and at the right speed. The pain was excruciating. For a few seconds I could not see at all and was completely dizzy. It was as if someone had given me anesthesia. For a while, I forgot about the pain in my bones and I thought that the Magnificent was absolutely right. But the pain in my soul had not gone away—it had not even diminished. It reigned with the same force in my heart. I woke up in the morning, after about three hours of sleep, with a huge bump and a constant ache throughout my head. But it didn't matter. I had to exhaust all options.

I loved enormously all these people who were seeking my well-being, and I had to follow their advice. I felt so indebted to them. I had already made the mistake of not listening to Egret. I hadn't listened to her in due time and had allowed the cancer to spread too much.

37

The One Who Saw It So Well

THE DAYS passed quickly, and on the twenty-first day I had to be back at the hospital. I deeply wished that the twenty-first day would disappear from the calendar. At the hospital, in the familiar crowded lobby, I waited in line for my turn. I watched other people's faces. They were wrinkled with despair and suffering, but I could also see an almost obsessive desire to stay alive, no matter what. We were all alike. We clung to life with a fanatical force. In front of me sat an extremely thin and frail man. He could barely breathe, and he was so pale that one could say he might die at any minute. I wanted to do something to help him, but I was afraid. I did not want to make him feel uncomfortable or totally helpless. He looked strikingly like Fr. Arsenie Boca.[1] He was of a surreal beauty. I could not look into his eyes. The intensity of his gaze unsettled me. I quickly ran away from that place and went outside the hospital in a hurry, where, on a bench, my docile and patient husband was waiting for me.

[1] Fr. Arsenie Boca (1910–1989) was a priest-monk, spiritual writer, and artist who suffered persecution under the Romanian Communist regime. People come from all over Romania to pray at his grave, located at Prislop Monastery.

"My love, my love!" I called to him excitedly. "Come with me quickly to see Fr. Arsenie.... He's in the line for the doctor.... Come on, give me your hand quickly!"

My husband stood up and said calmly and ironically, "Well, sure, my love, you have such great virtues indeed. Of course you were found worthy of seeing Fr. Arsenie...."

When we arrived in front of the man, my husband remained speechless. We both looked at him in shock. Out of the blue, I burst into tears—a ravishing, devastating sob. I could not stop. As if urged by an inner voice, I looked up at that man, a man who was in total pain. Then, that man, staring into my eyes, said to me with the voice of an angel, "We have to give up this poisoning.... In any case, I will not return here." He stood up suddenly and left hunched over, and I never saw him again.

He was such a dignified man, such a beautiful soul! And that day I decided to stop chemo.[2] I deeply wanted to have the courage necessary to give myself completely into God's hands. I stopped despite the fact that our spiritual father advised me to stick to chemo and the doctor's advice.

I had no strength to continue. All I wanted was to be able to make a lousy soup to feed my five little children every day. Making that soup became for me the light at the end of the tunnel, the ideal of my life. They loved it so much. They were all crazy for the soup made by their mommy. I prayed to St. Nektarios not to cure me from cancer, but to give me a little strength to cook for my children. Anyway, I had not

---

[2] As will be seen shortly, this would only be a temporary decision.

been requesting a cure, as I didn't believe one was possible.... Instead, I begged for a little strength for myself and mercy for my children.

Healing seemed a miracle too overwhelming for me. One day, my mother-in-law fell sick and became bedridden. Then I saw a glimpse of the amazing inner strength that could emanate from human endurance in the face of suffering. She had been blind for at least ten years. She was a woman of rare refinement, distinguished, elegant, and dignified. For the three months that I had to take care of her, I stopped chemo. I could not wash her or change her diapers if I had that devastating nausea. So, I stopped chemo, feeling inside that I had a really good reason for it. I was so proud. God won't allow me to die now, I thought. The mother of my husband, who is seventy-four, needs me so badly. I was bargaining with Him.

She waited docilely and patiently for me to bring her food. Most of the time I would run late, but she never complained. She would say to me, "May God give you health, Mioara. And pray, pray to God to keep your mind sane!"

At first I did not understand why she insisted so much on my mental sanity. Only after I lost her did I realize how right she was. I miss her so much. I miss her calm and gentle voice, her wrinkled and restless hands, which strongly gripped mine. She encouraged me so much.... "You'll be fine, you'll see." I don't have even a quarter of her dignity in the face of death. Toward the end of winter, we buried her, and once she was gone I lost a pillar of support in my life. No one could hug me and comfort me so beautifully.

She died as beautifully as she lived. In her blindness, she

taught me to clearly see my shortcomings and cowardice. I had made a huge mistake by not telling her how much I loved her.

She had made me see so well, but this would not last for very long. By March, I could not breathe anymore, and I obviously had to go back to the hospital. My doctor, now used to my disappearances, received me again under her protective wing. She was so understanding with Viorel and me. Each time we went to see her, my husband told her the stories invented by Justina and I smiled, not wanting her to see that I could barely breathe. One morning, everyone in the hospital was talking only about one thing, something that amazed them. It was all about …

38

The Doctor's Eyelashes

ONE DAY, I went for treatment. The doctor was an amazing woman. She did not wear any makeup, and her modesty put you at ease when she was around. I watched her blink with her new long and black eyelash extensions that made her face so sweet. She looked like a deer. She was beautiful anyway, but that day she was radiating a loveliness and delicacy that was simply stunning. My husband went to the seventh floor to pick up my sick-leave note. All that the people from that floor were talking about was the doctor's eyelashes. "I saw them myself," my husband confirmed confidently. "I would tell her they look great, but I don't know if that would be appropriate. I don't want her to feel offended."

"No, I would not advise you to say anything. Anyway, she does have great eyelashes," concluded the accountant, who was also in the office.

All the other doctors knew. All the janitors would lurk, waiting for the moment when the doctor would leave her office. As if nothing else mattered: neither the disastrous economic situation in Cyprus, nor the high levels of radiation from Fukushima. Even cancer cells would probably react differently when those amazing eyelashes were around. She

THE DOCTOR'S EYELASHES

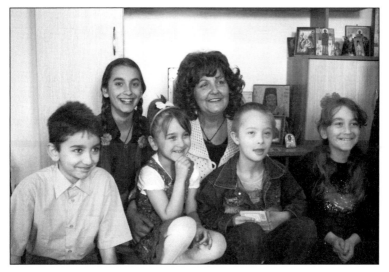

Mioara and children, April 9, 2014. Photo by Dinu Lazăr.

smiled rarely, but when she did, it felt like she was giving me undeniable hope.

I decided to go with Maria, my eleven-year-old daughter, to buy a wig. I couldn't have done it without her. She had an amazing aesthetic sense. "Dear, it's time to change your style.... I want to have a beautiful young mother." I was not young anymore, and much less healthy and beautiful, but she saw me in her own way.

"Hey, why are you crying?" she asked me one evening, finding me hidden outside the house.

"No, my doll, I'm not crying," I said quickly, drawing a fake smile on my face, "I got something in my eye."

"You know, Mommy, I wasn't born yesterday," she replied with a slight frown. "Please, take it easy. Otherwise, I'll call

Daddy, because I don't think you can afford to be depressed right now, when you have five children and a sick eighty-two-year-old mother to take care of."

Indeed, my mother had become seriously ill. For months she was not eating, and she was crying all the time. We brought her to our home. My mother was a former worker at the railway company. With an incredible inner strength she had faced mountains of hardships and problems throughout her life. She didn't have much schooling, but she possessed a depth and clarity of thought that I would not have been able to gain even if I had graduated from a hundred colleges. I knew she suffered a lot because of me. Three months before, in a moment when I could hardly breathe, I had begged her in a pretty serious tone, "I beg you, after I die, give charity to the poor in my memory!"

My Mom had her hands in her lap, fidgeting restlessly, and she said with tears in her eyes, "You won't die of cancer; you'll die of too much stupidity!"

Her words bewildered me. She had the great quality of capturing the very essence of things. She had read me, she had guessed my essence, she had put me into words so simply and deeply at the same time. I looked at her. Many years ago, two moles had broken out on her temple. After some time, that area festered and became like a little crater in her head. I thought I could almost see her brain if I looked through it. However, even with a hole in her head my mother was working all day long with an incredible vitality. I took her to the hospital. They set up a drip and gave her some pills, which my mother threw out the window at night. She defeated her skin cancer. She was forty when the doctors told her that she had only a few weeks left. She didn't listen to them. She was now eighty-two. But if my mother had literally had a hole in her head, I for one, had holes in my head and in my soul. Holes, lumps, and water in my lungs. This water did not want to go away. But I was not having it mechanically removed, either. It was like being in a boxing match.... The truth was that cancer had cornered me, and now it was bashing me with blows.

39

The Courage of Youth in the Face of Death

I WENT again to the hospital. I was waiting in line for the doctor. When I was I able to catch my breath, it felt like heaven. My leg shook frantically but I did not want to sit down. To me, this would have felt like giving up. I looked around. For the last two years I had been waiting in that hallway, and only then did I notice it: next to the doctor's office was another door on which there was a sign with a skull that read "Do not enter." I thought that perhaps one could get electrocuted in there. I asked myself rhetorically, "Why didn't I do this instead of two years of chemo?"

Compared to my fight with cancer, electro shocks seemed as smooth and light as a breeze of wind.

I observed the skull carefully. He looked like me. Just as bald and stupid. He looked at me reproachfully with his large, black, and deep eye holes. "What are you still doing here?" the skull seemed to ask me.

"Excuse me, could I go in before you?" a young voice brought me back to reality. "I'll be only a minute. I just want to ask if they have anything new for me…. You see, they experiment with new treatments on me, but they've exhausted all options, and I still have no chance to live. But who's to blame? If this is what God wants, I submit. I've lived for twenty-four years and I'm thankful for them."

I felt a terrible pity and I was ashamed to look at him. He had given me a great life lesson. There we were, in that line in a hospital corridor, women of all ages and of all colors, arranged, dyed, trimmed, wearing makeup, smiling hopefully, determined to reach a hundred years of age at least; women who did not want in any way to give up life, no matter how much they would be tortured. With no hair, no breasts, irradiated or poisoned, with one or more organs removed, it didn't matter how; it was important to live, to breathe a piece of life, a piece of time. We were more or less hypocrites, happy deep down that at least we with an incredible inner strength were not yet in the position of the twenty-four-year-old man, at the last boundary between life and death. I suddenly felt dizzy. My desperation to live caused me a state of anxiety, a terrible shame and nausea. I felt the need to sit down; I felt the need to embrace that man with all my strength. He seemed like he had come from another world, a world that did not know the fear of death. I realized, though, that my gesture of embracing him would be inappropriate ... or maybe not.... I felt an urge to ask him to forgive me because I could not help him, because I didn't know how to have his detachment in the face of death. He seemed such a free young man. It was as if he glowed, almost aggressively free.

That day, after hours of waiting in front of the doctor's office, I realized that it was useless for me to enter. It seemed like nonsense to fight desperately for my life at forty-seven when nothing could be done for a man in his twenties.

And all those children suffering from all kinds of cancers in hospitals ... all those angels.

O God! Their eyes ... as if they had been through all the wars in the world.

I remember how, that same day, I saw in the same line a gorgeous bald boy with many cuts on his head, probably from brain tumor operations. He was no more than five or six. He was waiting with his mother for X-rays of his lungs. He looked at us. It wasn't curiosity in his eyes, but rather a certain maturity, empathy, and understanding of our suffering. At one point, he laid his eyes on my husband, who had a long white beard. Perhaps the boy thought that my husband was Santa Claus. My husband couldn't bear that gaze and lowered his eyes. The boy had the eyes of someone who had lived an entire life. It was too much for one day. The young man, now this boy, the fragility of their age ... A fragility that somehow strengthened us older ones so much.

Their suffering woke me up from a long and surreal nightmare. I remember how that day I waited until everyone had left, until only my husband and I remained. We were sitting on two cold chairs, staring somewhere in front of us blankly.... We both felt so alone and helpless ... so helpless.

I suddenly burst into tears. I burst like a torrent, like a late autumn storm. Viorel, exasperated every time I cried, told me, "If you cry, I'll go home. You know, I can't bear it anymore! Look, I even got you a book by the Holy Fathers about depression."

THE COURAGE OF YOUTH IN THE FACE OF DEATH

Through hiccups and tears, I looked at the book. It was called *How to Heal Depression*. I browsed through it briefly. While reading from it, I cried even more. I read and I cried … I cried and read. My husband became more desperate. "Well, if not even the Holy Fathers can calm you down, I don't know what else to do."

Upset, he went out. I remained alone. I was not thinking of my lung metastases anymore. It was all the same to me; they could multiply if they wanted. What I cared about now were the metastases of that young man, of all those hospital patients who were trying to survive one more day, one more second, who were trying desperately to freeze time, to keep the cancer cells under control. I cried for all people with cancer. I cried for the entire history of out-of-control metastases, from their origins to the present. I cried for all doctors, who for dozens, even hundreds of years had struggled with these crazy and uncontrollable cells. I cried for all children with cancer, and I cried for my husband, who, in a more or less conscious way, I had made go crazy. I would have carried on crying if at some point a man in his sixties had not sat in front of me. He was shaking and I thought he was sick.

"Have you just had your chemo? Do you feel dizzy?" I asked him, concerned.

"No, Ma'am," he said, hiccuping. "I'm going now to receive my treatment. But before, I took a sip of courage … you know, to warm up…."

Only then I noticed the persistent sour smell of stale booze in the air.

"So ... you're on chemo and you still got drunk.... Aren't you feeling nauseous?"

"Ah, no, because after chemo I'll have a refreshing beer.... And now, before the nurse calls me in, I'm going to have a cigarette," he said, and he winked.

I loved him so much at that moment.

He represented life in all its brutality, instinct, and beauty. I would have embraced him regardless of that smell of poor booze. How could he bear it all? What was keeping him alive? What mechanism had his brain unlocked to cope with chemo, booze, and cigarettes, all at the same time?

I felt so powerless. Out of the twenty-one days between the chemo sessions, for about seventeen I could barely swallow water.... I would actually throw up even water. My body would not tolerate anything. I tried everything: tea, juices, water with lemon, even beer.... It was all useless. Until one day, when I discovered something I could easily swallow, that slid down my throat like magic and, by some miracle, I did not throw up. I found something that my body accepted and moreover liked, loved, and assimilated. That something was actually ...

40

My Tears and "Ovid's Tears"

I DISCOVERED it at a monastery, while we had lunch. I said to myself, "I'll just taste a little." I had had my chemo just two days before, and I felt nauseous from my brain to my liver. My lips and tongue burned. "Taste just a little, Mommy," Anthony said. "It's the famous wine Ovid's Tears. It undergoes two kinds of special treatment, and it's kept in 500-liter oak containers." Initially I tasted only a few drops, being used to throwing up everything. Nothing happened. I tasted some more—I still did not vomit. The miracle happened right before my eyes in its entire splendor. I managed to drink half a glass. I was so dehydrated that I felt the wine fly through my veins with a sharpness and clarity that was hard to describe in words. I could almost hear it reviving me, as if it were my primordial blood, my way of being and existing. Its aroma made me feel so alive. I slowly felt the desire to fight growing in me again. I felt that with this wine I could annihilate any toxicity in this world. I had the acute feeling that huge branches were growing in my veins, with their roots deeply embedded in my immune system. I felt how my whole immune system had become, in fact, a huge, solid, green tree, with roots watered by "Ovid's tears."

I drank another half a glass. I felt a slight dizziness and a sweet drowsiness. I felt the tree branches going not only through my veins but also to my brain. All of a sudden, I became very brave, and I felt I could fight a whole mountain of malignant cells.

My red cells had become adamant rocks. I was not afraid anymore of CT scans or of inches of water in my lungs.

When we got home, I went to the first supermarket to buy a bottle of the famous wine. It was rather expensive. I felt guilty.… "Should I buy it or not?" I remembered that tipsy man I had met the week before in the hospital. I understood him so well. "My brother, where are you to see me now?" Only then did I realize that I must not judge lest I be judged.

My survival instinct filled me completely. I had been so dehydrated for months that I could not resist the temptation, and eventually I bought the wine.

Each time I drank it, I felt new perspectives and new horizons opening in front of me.

At school the teacher told the children, "Write down the sentence 'My mother drinks water.'"

Justina replied, "But my mommy doesn't drink water, she drinks wine."

The class went quiet. The teacher was in a true existential dilemma.

At home, while enjoying the "tears," my own tears started to flow again. I thought in horror that if the cancer won't get me, then the drinking will. I saw myself swallowed by hell.

It was a cold autumn afternoon, and it was just Viorel and me at the kitchen table. I was drinking wine, he was drinking chamomile tea. It seemed unfair to change roles so suddenly. Determined to get out of this spell that was controlling me, I asked my husband to let me have some of his "same old boring chamomile tea." I took a few sips. Everything was back to normal. I threw up immediately and violently. Only then did I recognize myself. Only then was I again the real me. Only then did I remember that I was poisoned. I could not remember how it was to be healthy. I couldn't remember a life without chemo.

But maybe it was better that way.... Whenever I tried to run from the cross, it got worse. It hurt terribly that for Justina I had become "the mommy who drinks wine." This idea terrified me. And yet, this Ovid's Tears was so good, so sweet, and so alive. It made me so brave for a moment.

It gave me something that I had sought my entire life: courage, the courage to be myself, the courage to accept myself as I was.

41

The Architecture of Sacrifice

I WAS in church with my children. During the service, I told them that I needed a bit of water, and I went outside the church and cried. I could not do it inside. I felt like someone was looking at me and I felt ashamed. I went behind a corner of the church and fell to my knees begging for the mercy of the Virgin. Just then I felt a strong hand on my shoulder and a voice asked if I needed help. History repeated itself. I had nowhere to cry. At home the children saw me, at church those wonderful people saw me, and at the hospital my husband saw me.

It was a cool spring Sunday. After the service, a lady who was an architect called me outside in order to help me with an herbal remedy for strengthening my immune system.

I looked at her dazed. She was so young and beautiful that I wondered when she had time to learn so much and especially to have three children.

Her beauty and vitality were almost too much. She gave me some pills. By only looking at them I felt a bit stronger. They were like little bombs in me. The architect had a strong sense of values. She didn't seem to be affected by any of the vanity of this world. She built a new foundation for my soul.

"Mioriṭule,[1] leave everything behind.... You're not sick with cancer, but with worries.... Take the icon of the Virgin Mary and cover it with tears."

"Well, I can't breathe.... It's hard.... I can't even make soup." I tried to argue in favor of my despair.

"Well, hello!" responded the architect with an imperturbable calm. "Forget about worry. Smile, pray, relax, walk ... Come on, let's get together...."

God, how I loved her! She taught me how to grab life by the throat, how to detach myself from worries, and how to think. When I heard "Mioriṭule," I felt my tumor markers being lowered instantly. I don't know if she will ever realize what she really did for my soul. It hurt me so much that I had nothing to give her, until one evening, when praying, I heard Macrina saying, "Lord, thank you for giving Miha to us, to take care of our mother!"

By this "giving" I realized that our love was all we could ever give her. The love of my children for her was and would be our only gift to her.

---

[1] A diminutive for Mioara.

42

Disabled from Yesterday to Forever

THE DAYS were fleeting, just like the air in my lungs. I panted at almost every step. I had exhausted almost all the types of chemo and treatments. I did not know what to do to keep my right lung breathing. The left one seemed alive, breathing, but it did not help too much. It felt like a ton of rocks pressed on my right lung each time I inhaled. And each time I exhaled, I felt as if I were pulling wagons of scrap iron. But it was still good. My children could see me every day, and their hunger for their mother was satisfied. Meanwhile we decided to apply for disability benefits. Any extra penny would have helped us a lot. I had to go in front of a commission, which would decide whether I was disabled enough to qualify for the benefits. In the lobby of an old, creepy building, there were dozens of people: one-handed, blind, paralytic, as if that lobby were a valley of tears. Everywhere there were wheelchairs with paralyzed people.

The air smelled like ailments, helplessness, and despair.

Most of them had resigned expressions, devoid of any trace of hope. That was the most depressing part.

At the last CT scan, they had given me no more than three months left to live. But that was not what hurt me the most. It was the pain of my loved ones, the pain of my children. I started to understand those disabled people so well, their beautiful souls trapped in those crippled bodies.

That day my husband had told me off for dressing so ugly. I was wearing a pair of old pants, a loose t-shirt, and a knitted hat on my head. Given how ravaged my soul was, I did not care how I looked on the outside. My husband instead was wearing a suit and a tie. After hours of waiting, we entered a half-lit room. At a table there were three ladies busily writing something in some big files.

One of them looked at me through her glasses, and asked me, "So, Ma'am, what is your husband's disability?"

I was speechless with astonishment. I looked poor, pale, shabbily dressed, lost, and yet, despite my appearance, three doctors specializing in assessing various types of disability considered me "normal." This gave me unbelievably huge hopes. I remained silent.

"Hey, lady, I asked you what your husband's disability is?"

"Doctor," my husband answered, visibly annoyed, "I have a permanent disability, but I do not want to say which one."

His words caused a small uproar in the office. I quickly jumped in, trying to explain and to apologize for his sarcastic remark. "You know, I'm the disabled one. I don't have a breast, I can't use a hand, I don't have a lung, and to be honest I don't have much air, either."

Only then, after looking again in their files, did they realize that my husband was the normal one. They approved

CANCER, MY LOVE

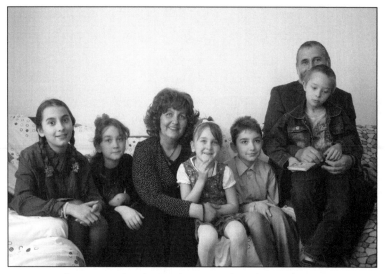

The Grigore family, April 9, 2014. Photo by Dinu Lazăr.

my benefits, and we quickly left that room, that lobby, that building, and those suffering people with various disabilities. It seemed like escaping a battlefield.

Only then did I realize how brave disabled people were. Seeing them there had given me something that enriched me, that made me think differently. I loved all those people who were disabled just like I was.

So, from that day on, in our household there were three officially disabled people—my mother, Nektarios, and myself—as well as one person only suspected of being disabled: my husband.

43

From Vienna to Bucharest

ONE MORNING, my husband, desperate to keep me alive, told me almost feverishly, "I've made an appointment with the best specialist from Vienna. He comes to Bucharest once a month and we'll show him your CT scan. It's impossible for him not to find a solution.... You can talk to him for thirty minutes, and it will cost us about 8 million lei."[1]

The truth was that 8 million for half an hour seemed quite a lot. I could have bought so many things for my children with that money. The day of the appointment finally came, and we arrived at the practice of this famous doctor. There were only wealthy people waiting. The air smelled of foreign and expensive perfumes.

Everything was clean and shining. The impression given by his practice was one of opulence and professionalism. I had all my five children with me. I was dressed like a peasant, with a skirt, a traditional blouse, and a scarf wrapped around my head. When the guards saw us they wouldn't let us inside the clinic. We explained that we actually had an appointment, and they asked if we had the money to pay for the medical

---

[1] At that time, this was about 250 dollars, or 180 euros.

examination. That made us feel so humiliated. We offered to pay in advance. They eventually let us go in, but then we caused another fuss in the lobby because the nurses panicked when they saw all our five children coming in with us. They were concerned that they might be noisy and disturb the famous doctor.

Although they were all seated, almost frozen with fear, the nurses made a wall around them, afraid that one might escape and rush into the office to disturb the doctor. My husband and I went inside and had a brief dialogue about the history of my cancer. There was another doctor translating, but I managed to tell him directly in English what an amazing husband and children I had. The doctor looked puzzled; he shook his head and asked for my last CT scan. When he saw my lungs on the CT scan, he raised one finger up to the sky and said solemnly, "Only God, only God."

Well, I already knew that "only God ..."; my children knew that much as well. If I knew that it would cost me 8 million lei to learn something I already knew, that "only God" could save me, I would have rather given this money to a monastery or to some poor people.

Toward the end, when the thirty minutes to which I was entitled were coming to an end, with my cheeks burning with anger, the peasant in me felt like she could not take this charade any longer. I went out like a whirlwind, grabbed my children from the nurses, and brought them one by one into the doctor's office. Two guards came in quickly trying to get my kids out of the office. It was as if I had put a bomb near the Austrian doctor and not five small children. When they

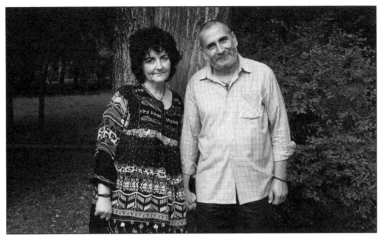

Mioara and Viorel.

wanted to take us out, the doctor made a sign to leave us, and we all stood in front of him.

"Look," I told him, "Macrina wants to become a painter, Justina dreams of being a ballerina, Anthony will be a scientist, Maria a poet, and Nektarios is our angel.... Don't you think I have enough reasons to fight to stay alive?"

At that, it seemed like the doctor's heart softened and he looked with love at all of us, confirming once again that a miracle from God was the only hope in my case.

"Only God, only God"—his words accompanied me to the door.

We went home. The drive back seemed long and tiring. There was nothing cooked at home, so I quickly boiled some potatoes. We fell asleep embracing, as usual.

I kept thinking about how stupid I was to put all my hopes in people and clinging to doctors and their promises as my only hope. I dreamed that my five children and I were wandering through Vienna, and in the evening we went to a concert at the State Opera. I knew it was one of the most important operas in the world. I was with my children and my husband in the third row. The heavy, thick, imperial curtain opened, revealing a large choir. The song, barely perceptible at first, became gradually more serious, more acute, until the chorus erupted like a volcano. I listened closely and I could not believe my ears.... The choir sang only one verse: Only God, only God.... All of their eyes were fixed on me, somewhat reproachfully. I woke up dizzy. The song followed me throughout the day.... Only God, only God. I had to go all the way to Vienna in my dream, to realize that all I had left was God, that only God was my first and my last frontier.

44

The Long Way of Innocence

I OFTEN saw him in church. He was tall and thin, wearing his hair in a ponytail. He had the innocent expression of a child. Moreover, he was funny and almost unbearably smart. He was around thirty and many girls wanted him around. They swarmed around him like bees around a flower, but he was more or less absent-minded, apparently distant. He seemed to live in a world where only children were allowed.

He was surrounded by children: big, small, poor, oppressed, orphans.... With whatever he earned he used to buy clothes and food for them. One day he came to our house, and he taught our children to play again, to laugh out loud, and to see beyond doctors, disease, and hospitals.

One day, he took Justina in his arms and said, "I'm condemned to love you forever." He had a power of sacrifice and dedication to children, beyond any limit of understanding.

"Come on, let's play!" and all my five children, with tremendous joy, surrounded him with their arms and began playing nice and sweet childhood games. I looked at them and all my nausea disappeared as if by magic. I do not know if he will ever realize what he meant to me and to my children. I don't know if he will ever realize how much joy he gave me

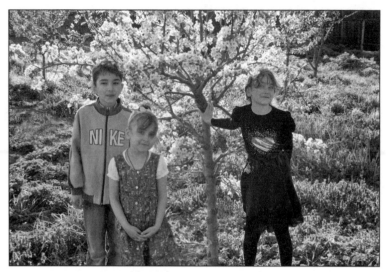

The Grigore children outside their home, April 9, 2014. Photos by Dinu Lazăr. *Above, left to right:* Anthony, Justina, and Macrina.

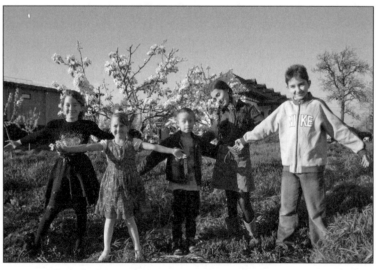

Left to right: Macrina, Justina, Nektarios, Maria, and Anthony.

when he brought us a huge juicy watermelon on that particular day when I was vomiting and my blood pressure was 8. I don't know if he will ever realize that his games gave back to my children the joy of playing together, of laughing out loud. Their joy meant the world to me.

And so, the days passed, and my children got a priceless friend, a friend who gave them what they had not received before: the gift of playing games, and through this, the joy of living.

He restored my children's lost youth.

Time passed. I didn't even need a calendar. I knew that on the day of the chemo, three weeks had already passed since my last hospital visit. Other than that, I continued to live in constant wonder and amazement. On Sundays, during the Holy Liturgy, I would stand by the door of the church, almost embarrassed to face those people who fought so hard for me. The people I loved, my heroes, would ask me every week how I felt … and they would hug me tightly.

"A true Christian does not desperately hold onto his life, but gives himself to God's will." The words of my spiritual father rang in my ears.

But I was held to this life by some invisible threads. I clung with all my being to X-rays, tomography, infusions. Where the right lung used to be the last X-ray showed a kind of fog, a steam, as if it were a bright and transparent cloud.

I could see myself floating in that cloud, freed from any trauma, any medical prognosis, or any scanner. I did not know if that light steam or cloud in my lung was water, or if it was devoured tissue. All I knew was that I could breathe less and

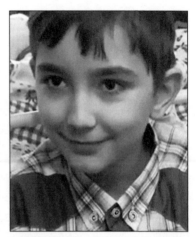

Photo stills from a video recorded in the Grigore home, April 2014. *Top right:* Anthony. *Middle left:* Macrina. *Middle right:* Justina. *Bottom, left to right:* the Grigore family praying before their icons. Maria, Macrina, Anthony, Justina, Nektarios, Mioara (in front of Viorel, holding Nektarios), and Viorel.

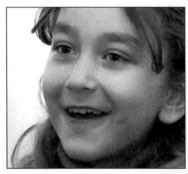

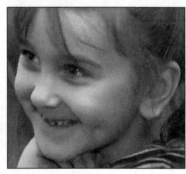

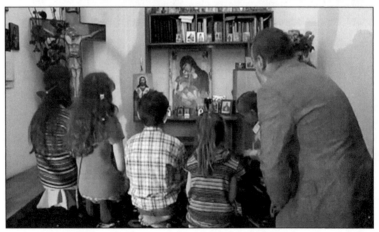

less. I felt devastated. But I still had something invaluable. The people around me.

What would I have done without Egret and her little wonder-pills, without her insistence and love? What would I have done without Aida and her engineer, without the architect and the new foundation she built in my soul? What would my kids have done without their friend, or how would I have lived without his joy and smile?

"This is how God holds you in His hands," said Joy one day, showing me the cupping of her hands. Her hands seemed to radiate thousands of rays of light.

Rays of light that prolonged my life and made me a partaker in the wonder of "still being here."

45

Mesopotamia Not Forgotten

SUDDENLY, my mother's illness worsened. She was agitated, crying all the time, with no appetite. She had lost about twenty kilos[1] in four months. She became quiet, withdrawn. She closed herself off in a world of her own where I had no access. I could not recognize her. It was as if I had six children. I took her to the hospital. I passed out in the hallway from the chemo. The doctors asked confusedly who the patient actually was. My mother's tests showed the health of a twenty-year-old person.

"It's something to do with stress," the doctor on duty told me. I could no longer communicate with her. That hurt tremendously.

She had been with me for so long. Even though she was alive, I felt like I was losing her, little by little, every day.

I was more and more afraid that if I died before her, there would be no one to take care of her. I did not know if Viorel would have the strength and the patience to take care of her after losing me.

My despair was directly proportional to the number of

---

[1] About forty-four pounds.

children in the house. As my mother became a child, my panic attacks increased every day. I would take her by the hand and take a daily walk with her through the garden. In fact she was walking me: the lack of air forced me to stop and sit down every ten minutes.

"Mom, my love, return to me. Be like I always knew you."

She looked through me. My tears were ready to burst out.

"I have such a big sadness," murmured my mother, at her venerable age of eighty-two. She was so beautiful. She was surreally slender, pale, with large blue eyes, as if the whole sky were reflected in them.

"What's upset you, my doll?" I asked, with my heart ready to jump out of my chest, as if I saw a glimpse of hope that she might return to normal.

"It hurts," my mother said, pausing as if for an eternity. "It hurts me that I can't remember the multiplication table. I forgot it in the third grade. I would not want to die without remembering it. Could you please teach me, pretty please?"

Her look and her voice continually begged me. We sat down among trees with rusty leaves in the autumn sun, and I began to recite for her the multiplication table.

After three decades or so since I had learned it, I was afraid I had forgotten it as well. As I was teaching it to her, I saw how her face lit up slightly with a smile. She was so happy, as if a huge burden had been taken from her soul. By the time I got to ten, my mother was at the peak of joy.

"Who invented the multiplication table, my doll?" she asked me with an unusual curiosity. It was as if her entire life depended on my answer.

Suddenly, my palms began to sweat. I didn't know what to answer, and that made me panic. Sweat covered my face.

"Anthony, Anthony!" I desperately ran inside the house. I felt that he was the only one who could help me quickly. He was in the yard chopping wood with his father.

"Who invented the multiplication table?" I asked him almost panting.

"Mom, how could you not know a thing like that?" Anthony replied, placing the wood near the wall of the house. "The Mesopotamians, of course. They invented numbers."

I returned to my mother in the garden and, clasping her hands in my hands, I told her with satisfaction, "Mom, the multiplication table was invented in Mesopotamia."

"I see …," my mother replied thoughtfully, as if the Mesopotamians would have solved the most difficult dilemmas of her life.

Evening was coming down over the trees of the garden. Everything seemed so tired and ephemeral.

At night, while everyone was asleep, I thanked God and the Virgin that my mother was still alive; that I, in my cowardice, was still alive to take care of her; and that I had managed not to mess up the multiplication table.

For the first time, I saw the beauty, harmony, and perfection of the multiplication table. I had never thought about how mysterious and harmonious it was. I felt an indefinable longing for the Mesopotamians. Thousands of years ago, they basically changed the lives of millions of people.… And I rediscovered them through my Mom, while multiplying my love for her.

46

Somewhere between a Broken Heart and the Majesty of a Mountain

I STILL remember: I was climbing and climbing without stopping, but the peak of that mountain seemed further and further away. It became something impossible to reach.... It was like the miracle of my healing, too overwhelming for me. I hadn't hiked in years. Besides, I knew that the fatigue and shortness of breath caused by the lung cancer would not allow me to climb a little hill, let alone a mountain. But I had to do it.... I had to overcome my own cowardice and great helplessness. I was tired of playing the victim. "Will I be able to do this? Will I be able to carry so much pain when the time comes to part with my children? Will I be able to climb that mountain before death gets me?"

What madness had possessed me to even think about hiking? I could barely climb a few steps, let alone a mountain. But I had to do it for the sake of the kids, for the sake of their love. I simply had to find the right place where I could explain to them that soon I would leave them. That soon I would go to another world, a world where maybe I would have the chance to love them in a different way, to pray for them, to feel and think differently, and not so possessively and selfishly as I had done in this world.

"Mommy, Mommy, we beg you, let's go to the mountains! We want that so much …," pleaded all my five children one morning.

As usual, my body was trembling. My knees, my feet, my heart. It was two weeks since chemo, and almost four years since I had started battling this terrible and at the same time noble disease. Cancer, my nightmare. Cancer, my love. Love for all those heroes in my life, all those people who had fought alongside me on the front lines and had felt together with me all the bullets of pain shredding their flesh.

The tanks of malignant cells had passed over them, but they still had not given up; they still resisted for me on the battlefield of my cancer.

That day, we arrived at the foot of the mountain around eleven in the morning. The cold air of a bitter winter made it almost impossible for me to breathe.

I covered myself with a long and thick scarf around my mouth, and we started to ascend.

At first slowly, gradually, with fear and caution, then a little faster.

After a few yards we stopped, because I felt like I could not go on.

I was breathing so heavily that my children flanked me on both sides and kept repeating, "Easy, Mommy, easy. Relax." I sat under a tree. It was the end of 2013. I felt it was also my end. I would be so happy to die climbing that mountain—to die climbing, and not descending like at the beginning of my life. Towards the end of my life, I wanted to climb and not fall. My entire life I had fallen.... I saw in my mind flashes of my life, pieces of time that simply melted without even my realizing how and why.

I thought about summer. I thought of my last CT scan when instead of the right lung there was only that fluffy and white cloud ... too white and too fluffy ... and I could not remove the doctor's words from my brain: "There is no chance, absolutely none."

O God! And I hadn't prepared my children for my departure.... I hadn't told them once and for all how much I loved them.

I remember that hot summer day, when I was given the last prognosis, which devastated me. I had gone home, and all I wanted to do was to take a shower.... I was feeling so dirty, so heavy and sinful.

The children were playing outside. There, in the small shower stall, perhaps too narrow for me, I felt I had no more air. I almost felt as if I were in the CT scanner. Thousands of chains were strangling my heart. For me, any narrow space was a piece of hell. I turned on the hot water. Although it was hot outside, the almost boiling water made me feel so good.

I could hear the voices and the laughter of my children outside. I thought desperately that the three months I had left to live would fly by, and my children would be left without their mommy suddenly and without any explanation. And they would run around the yard asking about their mommy, and my husband would not be able to make them understand. Understand what? What could we expect from a five-year-old girl or from a little boy with Down syndrome? How could we expect them to understand that God, in His great mercy towards me, had given me this disease as a last hope or as a last chance for my soul?

They were so hungry for their mother: to touch her, to bite her, to tickle her, to embrace her, to feel her tangibly and concretely next to them.

Hot water ran down my body and it had no effect on my frozen heart.

I was so sad and frozen that I felt the need to raise the temperature of the water even more. It got hotter and hotter ... until I suddenly realized the horror of the whole situation. I realized and saw clearly the hell inside my heart, that coldness which had frozen me and made me tremble for so long ... that coldness I had felt inside for years, that existential and overwhelming coldness.

And then, for the first time, I cried out ... I cried out to God, asking for forgiveness with all my frozen heart. I was naked in front of Him, both in body and in soul. "God, forgive me!" I cried out, falling to my knees while the ever hotter water burnt my back, hunched under so many sins. But I could no longer feel the heat. All I could feel was the boundless weight of my heart, which sadness had petrified. I yelled and howled for mercy and forgiveness to God and to His Most Pure Mother at such an undignified moment, at a time and place almost unthinkable: in a small shower stall. But it was there and then that I realized it was pointless, absolutely pointless, to survive and live near my children if I did not live first of all for and in God.

I do not know how long I cried, I do not know how long the hot water burnt my back, but that moment was for me a great release, a release for which I had been waiting my whole life.

Suddenly, I heard Justina shouting, "Help, help! Mommy is screaming in the bathroom!"

I stood up suddenly, almost mechanically, and, filled with shame, I got dressed quickly and went into the yard so that my children could see me.

We embraced with a crazy thirst and started running through the trees as if nothing had happened. I could not explain anything to them. I could not look into their eyes and tell them that I would die soon and they would never see me again. When I looked into their little eyes, I felt like fainting. They were so small and so many.

I was at the foot of the mountain. My heart rate had slowed down a bit. My children helped me stand up.

"It's okay, Mommy, we'll come back next year, if you can't make it now …," my children told me with compassionate voices.

"Next year, for sure we'll come again, all of us together, my love," my husband reassured me, as if he were giving me a coded message. "You won't die now, not now…. You'll continue to be with us."

But I knew, I felt, I was absolutely sure that I would not live for another year. So I decided to make a leap in time, and bring the following year to the present and somehow make this moment immortal.

So, we started to climb. My husband and my children were pulling me by my hands. My heart was racing. I felt as if my lungs would burst at any moment. I did not know what I could do in order to breathe a little better.

"Mom, Mom, did you know?" Anthony asked, while towing me like a wreck, too heavy and too big for him. "Did you know that in 1985 a cyclist named John Howard reached the incredible speed of 245.08 kilometers per hour, being helped by the slipstream effect of a race car driving in front of him, a car obviously modified?"

My thoughts flew immediately to all those brave and sacrificial people in my life, to all those who, like the slipstream effect of that race car, had breathed in my suffering with their love. I thought of the architect, who told me, "Mioriţule, we have to clean your liver now," but she had already cleaned my soul of so many fears and doubts. I thought of Egret, who constantly told me, "Don't worry, I'll love you with or without a brain, if the cancer goes there, too." I thought of Joy, who with each hug would crack not only my bones but also the metastases. "My fluffy sheep," she called me, as she touched my swollen hand with black nails smelling so bad and lifted it to her pale and clean cheek.

I felt as if the sky would fall down on me. I did not know how to repay them. I did not know how to return even a bit of the love they had given me, a love that seemed to dissolve all the poison from my veins.

I kept on climbing, but my knees were trembling so badly

BETWEEN A BROKEN HEART AND THE MAJESTY OF A MOUNTAIN

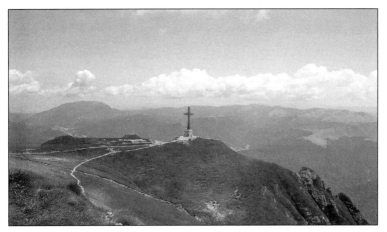

On this and the following pages: Views of the Heroes' Cross atop Caraiman Peak.

that I could not take another step, and I collapsed on some large rocks, hundreds of years old.

"Come on, my love, hang on," my husband said to me and he started to support me. He was so strong!

He pulled me more strongly than that race car. He seemed to me as strong and unshakable as that mountain we were climbing. The great cross was on the mountaintop.[1] The cross reigned over the mountain with dramatic majesty. It was my cross, the cross toward which I was climbing.

I remembered that tall gentleman from the church and his wife, who always beamed with joy. They had two gorgeous

---

[1] The Heroes' Cross is a monument built atop Caraiman Peak, at an altitude of 7,516 feet in the Bucegi Mountains of Romania. It is 118 feet tall, and is made out of steel, with a concrete pedestal clad with stone. Completed in 1928, it was consecrated on September 14 of that year, the Feast of the Exaltation of the Precious and Life-giving Cross.

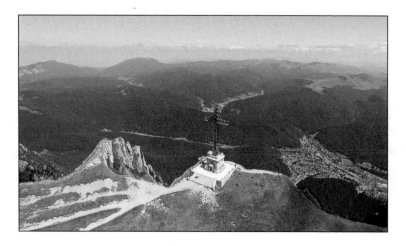

twin boys, about six, and a girl just as gorgeous. I was climbing and thinking of how beautifully they were raising their children, of how beautifully and sacrificially they helped me carry my cross. They were so gentle to give and sacrifice so much of themselves.

"Lord-Lord, please have mercy on the mommy of five little children," their little girl, who was only seven or eight, had once prayed for me at a monastery. Their innocence, their gentleness, their ability to feel the pain of their neighbor and to almost take it upon themselves melted my heart.

I climbed and I felt that I had no air at all left in my lungs. I felt my heart somewhere in my head, and the increasingly thin air sent thousands of needles throughout my whole body.

But at the same time I started to feel a certain joy and a new courage. My children's little hands pushed me from behind, and the strong hand of my husband pulled me after him with tremendous force.

My breathing became quick and difficult as I thought of

BETWEEN A BROKEN HEART AND THE MAJESTY OF A MOUNTAIN

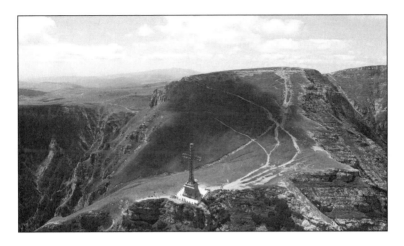

the childlike friend of my children's lives, of that "man-child," who restored their childhood by playing with them. The night before I had asked him, "Do you think I can rise to the occasion? I'm still so afraid of those awful pains of the last moments. I'm afraid I won't be able to bear them."

"The pains are behind; from now on the joys will come," that good and pure man answered me. In a second, he had given me huge wings. He had melted my fear with a just a few words.

I had not done anything to deserve the love, so unique and special, of these people.

I climbed and, through drops of sweat, I thought of another two wonderful young people, Andreea and Daniel, married only for a few years, who would teach us what love for one's country, love for the land of our ancestors, for our traditions, truly was. They worked in Bucharest, but every weekend they would return to their country house, to the place from where they were absorbing the power to live and love ... somewhere in Argeș, at Călinești.

When they came back to Bucharest, they would give us the most natural and best-tasting smoked cheese and the best buttermilk. Everything tasted so fresh and unaltered. The husband, Daniel, would tell my children how he was scything grass in the summer ... he was a true master of scything. He brought back into our lives that particular longing to fall in love again with our homeland.

I climbed, even though I felt I could not take one more step. I had no air. I sat down again under a tall pine and my children sat next to me. The air smelled of pine cones and of cold. I panted and thought of St. John Maximovitch from America, about whom I found out from a lady whose vitality and wisdom gave me strength to go on.... When I had seen her coming toward me with her face shining with optimism (she had a fantastic capacity to believe in the miracle of my healing), I had felt like my bones no longer hurt. I had never told her about the therapeutic effect she had on me.

I stood up and started to climb again. I did not know how long I would be able to go on. I felt like I would explode and millions of particles would spread from me, full of longing for, and gratitude toward, all these heroes of myself and of my children.

I climbed and looked at the cross. It was waiting for me patiently, as it had waited for me all my life. It had waited for me to embrace it with the joy of a true Christian.

I climbed and thought about my cancer. For the first time I accepted it, and for the first time I did not want to feel any fear of it. I was tired of fear, and of all the restlessness it caused.

My cancer was mine and only mine. It was part of my

being. Perhaps I was the cancer, but maybe I was too afraid to admit it. And maybe the cancer was scared of me too, because for so many years it had been hunted and harassed by me. For the first time I felt a terrible pity for all those sick cells, so stubborn to live.

If God allowed them to live in me, why wouldn't I love them? I had all these people around me who taught me how to love and especially how to sacrifice my ego—an ego as big as that mountain.

My legs would not hold me anymore.... Every step I took toward the cross was a won battle. Every step was actually one more mine neutralized.

Three children pushed me from behind, two pulled me by my left hand, and my husband by my right hand. I felt like I was flying with them. My entire body hurt me, my longing for them and their longing for me hurt me, too. I watched my husband, who dragged me to the cross with an almost supernatural determination. He did not want to be without his wife, without the mother of his children. I wanted to cry and tell him how much I loved him and how grateful I was for all his love, for these thirteen years of marriage ... thirteen years that seemed a hundred and thirty, thirteen hundred, an eternity.... His love kept me alive even without a breast, without a hand, without a lung, without the courage to truly live. His love almost shook that mountain, making it more accessible to me. While I climbed, I kissed the hands of my husband, the hands of my children, and—in my thoughts—the hands of the Savior, feeling enormously sorry that I had crucified Him so many times.

I felt I could not take another step. The air seemed to be all gone, and I crumpled slightly at the base of a tree. We stayed there, embraced for a long time. "I want to give you all my air," my husband said with tears in his eyes.

I could not answer. I just smiled.

I looked again at the cross on the mountaintop. My thoughts flew quickly to the branch that appeared in the latrine of my childhood, the branch that saved me when I was seven, the branch that had pulled me to life, to air, to light. I did not know why I hadn't died then. But then I looked at my five little children. Their eyes were begging me to hang on, to carry on breathing. I stood up and began to climb again ... little by little.... I was pulled toward the top by the power of the Cross, by the love of my husband and of my children.

"Glory to Thee, O Lord!" was all I managed to say; and for the first time I loved my illness, I loved my cancer, I loved my suffering, a suffering that now seemed to be woven with little threads of joy.

We climbed and climbed ... we climbed toward heaven ... we climbed toward salvation ... we climbed toward the Cross.

Epilogue

EDITOR'S NOTE: The following article was published a month after Mioara's repose, in *Familia Ortodoxă* [The Orthodox Family], April 2015 (no. 75) pp. 12–19. The first section was written by Anca Stanciu, the editor of the Romanian edition of *Cancer, My Love,* who appears as "Joy" in this book. The two interviews that follow were conducted by Raluca Tănăseanu (not to be confused with "Dr. Raluca" in this book). Both Anca and Raluca are among the editors of *Familia Ortodoxă*.

I.

Mioara, My Love

by Anca Stanciu

SOME OF the most beautiful words on love I've ever heard were said by Fr. Sophrony Sakharov. They were repeated to me by Fr. Nikolai, his nephew. Interpreting Psalm 109 (110), *Sit Thou at My right hand, until I make Thine enemies Thy footstool,* Fr. Sophrony asked, "How? By force?" And he himself answered, "No. By love."

As a power that changes the world—first us, and wondrously those around us as well ("Acquire love, and thousands around you will be changed")[1]—love is a "weapon," the only

---

[1] A paraphrase of the well-known saying of St. Seraphim of Sarov (1759–1833): "Acquire the Spirit of peace, and thousands around you will be saved."

one with which our Lord and God Himself teaches us to do battle: *Love your enemies, bless them that curse you, do good to them that hate you, and pray for them which despitefully use you, and persecute you* (Matt. 5:44). Through love Christ responded to those who persecuted Him, through love He ascended the Cross, through love He destroyed death and conquered hell— a conquest that has taken place unceasingly in our souls from then unto this day.

As true Christians and followers of Christ, we know these things and practice them constantly in our lives. Therefore, we give our cloak to the one who wants to take our coat, and to the one who smites our face we turn the other cheek. Thus, our ears are not injured by a raised voice; words and feelings of hatred, strife, envy, slander, and judging do not trample down our souls; we haven't heard about divorces or poorly raised children in our midst, or about disobedience or revolts. Because we have love. And love has a power that changes the world: us first, and then those around us.

Don't you believe? Don't you believe in the Gospels?

Then listen. I will tell you a story. A never-ending story.

Behind the funeral bier a woman is mightily lamenting. It is an authentic lamentation, springing from an irrepressible pain: "My Miorița,[2] my child, don't go there.... Stay with me longer, and I'll care for you!"

There's a festal atmosphere despite the fact that it's a funeral. Nevertheless, almost none of us can suppress our tears

---

[2] A diminutive for Mioara.

EPILOGUE

as we listen to her. We proceed, more and more startled and shaken. Viorel approaches me and grabs my hand, "Do you see her? She mourns Mioara the most. Some think she is her mother. But no one knows.... She's the woman who took care of her during her last months.

"You wouldn't believe this woman had been stealing from our house. I would get very angry seeing this. But Mioara would always tell me, 'Let her, let her …' The next day [she would steal] again. Mioara would say again: 'Viorel, let her …' I would get vexed. 'Well, how am I going to let her? You'll see what I'm going to do to her!' 'Let her …'

"This kept going on until one day this woman fell at Mioara's feet in tears: 'Mioara, I've stolen from you.... I've slandered you … terribly! Forgive me.' Mioara was crying, too, embracing her. What repentance this woman had! Without us saying even a word to her …"

Sit Thou at My right hand, until I make Thine enemies Thy footstool. "By force?" "No. By love."

… Now do you believe in the Gospels?

* * *

We are not going to write a biography of Mioara here. She already wrote one, descending to the most hidden spots of her soul, in *Cancer, My Love:* a book that has captured an impressive number of amazed readers. Some feared reading it: could it be contagious? Others simply did not like the title: "This is inadmissible! It's … a pleonasm … an oxymoron, a stylistic device!" For yet others—the majority—reading the book has been a life-changing experience. It revived them; it helped them confront themselves and those dark corners that all of us try to hypocritically hide from ourselves and God. It brought some to the Faith and healed others of hidden fears. It comforted those in pain. Mioara's book was, for most of us, a mechanism that let loose a lever in our rusted hearts. It taught us to laugh and sob again with all our strength, and, above all, to love, to care about someone outside of our own precious selves.

Of course, you understand that the title reveals a certain spiritual level. Mioara attained love of enemies. Is there a greater enemy than the one killing you slowly but surely, in unbearable torments? Mioara loved this enemy that would change her life completely, that would shake and cast down every bit of the wall she had erected in her relationships with God and with her family—this enemy of which we fear even to hear its name. How—I ask you—how did she succeed?

I received the answer the day before her repose.

Because Mioara had become entirely love.

* * *

On Sunday, March 1, we learned she was feeling very poorly; therefore, we were afraid even to go to see her. We had visited her two weeks prior, and we had talked together for a long time. She had told us about the second volume of her book, which she had already sketched—in her mind!—during the sleepless nights of the past month. She was out of breath. Her lungs were not helping her anymore; they had shrunk very much, and thus her heart was beating very strongly to compensate for the lack of oxygen. It was as if she were constantly

EPILOGUE

running, day and night, or as if she were at a very high elevation, where the air was getting thinner and thinner....

We tried to visit her later on, but Viorel did not allow us. We understood she was feeling poorly—but how many times had she not been ailing before? How many times had she been given only two weeks to live? And every time Mioara would have a turnaround from death, with the same childish smile. It had to be the same this time too, no? She's feeling poorly but it will pass, right?

We went in to bring her a *mărțișor*.[3] She was happy to see us. She was changed. Terribly weakened—but I'm not referring to such a change. She had something we had not seen previously. She had an inner reconciliation. We no longer perceived the turmoil we had seen all those years before: "Ah, I'm dying ... ah, the children ...." Mioara was at peace.

Her every gesture during this last visit concealed a spiritual state.

We gave her the *mărțișor*. She suddenly became anxious: "And I ... I have nothing to give you...." She sent one of the children to bring us flowers, despite our resistance.

I knelt at the side of the bed, kissing her hand. She took my head and embraced it strongly, kissing me on the forehead. If I could have, I would have severed a part of me....

"Mioara, what can I give you? My lungs ... my heart ... my life?"

"You've already given me everything."

---

[3] A *mărțișor* is a red and white string with hanging tassel customarily given on the 1st of March, the celebration of Mărțișor (a diminutive for "March"), which in Romania marks the beginning of spring.

"Now you're going to get well, you'll see!" I told her with all my conviction. She was connected to an oxygen machine. "See, this oxygen enters your lungs, and the lungs will inflate now...."

She laughed then, she laughed mightily. It was amazing for a person so weak. For the first time she did not believe me, or she was not able to show that she believed me. She knew, this time she already knew. In my naïveté I remained puzzled.

Upon our departure she told us, "I love you.... I love you...."

Mioara had become love. Her words continue to have power.

I heard those words the next day also — they were still there, in the same house where now Mioara was deeply silent. A deep silence is a deep prayer, right? I was reading the Psalter at her head, and I felt that embrace she had given me with all her strength the day before. Such an embrace, of a person so weak, revealed precisely the power of her prayer: absolute. I was struggling to love her the same way, but alas, how insignificant I felt in the torrent of her love!

My beloved, if I ached from something it was because I was not able to respond to you with the same measure of love. I was a barren fountain, but you, a sea.... You called me "Joy" — ah, how well you deceived me! So many years! I saw now, at your bedside, that you are the Joy. But don't worry, you'll see, you'll see when we'll meet, you're not going to fool me the second time: when you shout: "Joy!" I will reply on the spot knowingly, "No, it's you! No, it's you!"

EPILOGUE

2.

"Mioara Gave Me the Chance of
Sanctification through Her Life"

An Interview with Viorel Grigore

Viorel, how were Mioara's last days?

They were very difficult, nightmarish days, of a harsh battle to prolong her life a few more moments, to take another breath.... Very difficult, and with tremendous suffering that cannot be expressed in words. But, towards the end of this battle, Mioara was able to go to the Lord with a certain serenity and peace, which is something extraordinary for us as a family and for me as a husband.

She knew these moments were numbered. She even told me, on the morning of her departure, that she didn't have much longer—but she didn't insist on this point, and allowed the children to go to school, being all in all at peace, and not lamenting much, as one in such pain would do. The pains were intense, but very much hidden and inhibited, so as not to frighten the children and us. In fact, she had become so weak that she was barely able to move. She told me the end was near and to take care of the children, to tell them stories and take them on walks....

You've told us of the physical battles Mioara endured, but how about the spiritual warfare?

The spiritual warfare was, comparatively, much more intense, more deceiving, more persistent.... Only she knew how fierce it was, because here lies the entire battle of man—whether contemporary or not: the battle with thoughts, which can isolate you and take you either to hell or to heaven. In this we had great help from our spiritual father, Fr. Arsenie of Cornu Monastery,[4] who guided us in this warfare in which the enemy is unseen and works on thousands of battlegrounds. One has to greatly persist in prayer. Sometimes you can hardly even pray, "Lord, have mercy!" or, "Lord!" or something else to take your mind away from the thoughts that come from the enemy and drive you crazy. Yet Mioara would basically cut off such thoughts through prayer: "Lord Jesus Christ …," "Most Holy Theotokos …"

Are there things others have told you about Mioara that have impressed you?

There are tens and hundreds of things that impress me about Mioara, and I hope all these things will be noted in the second book. I even promised her that I'll also write a book, and she even asked me to do it. I explained to her that I don't have this gift, but that if she's going to pray for me from heaven, maybe I'll write a book, with Maria's help. There I'll tell everything she did before the wedding and after; it's a pretty packed and very unusual biography.

There were people present at the funeral who did not know Mioara before. Why do you think all these people came?

They didn't know Mioara, [but they came] because she was renowned through her book. I found myself in the midst of people I had never seen in my life. On the first day of the

[4] Fr. Arsenie Muscalu is the father confessor of the Monastery of St. John the Evangelist and the Holy Virgin Euphrosyne in Cornu, Prahova County.

EPILOGUE

wake, a woman showed up bringing me some gifts. "You don't know me," she said, "but I know Mrs. Mioara. I've read her book and I want to give the children some gifts. You don't have to care about what my name is or who I am"—and she disappeared....

What was the atmosphere like at the funeral?

It was a miracle, because during the entire wake and before the funeral the weather was bad, cold, rainy, windy, and stormy, but at the funeral the weather was superb, sunny. So, even if viewed only from this perspective, she was seen to be greatly loved by God. All the people present, even the Fathers,[5] felt a peaceful ambience, not as if you were next to a corpse. I had the same feeling, although I hadn't felt the same when I stood by my father's and mother's bodies. It was something indescribable.

How do you feel Mioara now?

I feel her very happy, and that's why I rejoice and give glory to God that I was by her side until she went to the next life. I believe with complete confidence that she is in her place, where she is doing very well.

From which of her virtues did you benefit the most?

I think I mostly benefited from her great patience, enduring the evil your neighbor can do to you, which he or she commits ceaselessly. I would not have resisted such shocks, I would have reacted somehow, but she did not react. She was patient. She gave the second and the third and the thousandth

---

[5] These included priests and deacons, and the priest-monk who was Mioara's spiritual father, the above-mentioned Fr. Arsenie Muscalu of Cornu Monastery.

chance, and all these things bore fruit. It's very hard to find such a person.... In the end, it's part of the humility of a true Christian.

She had another virtue also: she was very merciful. At some point, when she was in a lung hospital in Bucharest, she met a family of two young people who were struggling with a merciless illness that had no diagnosis at that point. He had been caring for his wife for about three years; they were both very young, and Mioara helped them with some money and advice. That man was very surprised by Mioara's gesture, knowing that her own situation was not the best—even worse than his wife's. But Mioara had a remarkable strength that enabled her to prevail at a time when you consider yourself condemned in the face of death. In fact, she fought tremendously, for the children and for the love of God first of all. To the last moment, she did not give up. She had a great ability to sacrifice herself, and had extraordinary courage.

Many spoke of her great love for people ...

Yes, she had an immense love for people. She loved her neighbor more than she loved herself. She was able to give some of her organs just so that another might have a beam of joy on his countenance. I only realized this later, but I had an amazing opportunity in the life we had together, which I believe was a great miracle. Mioara gave me the chance of sanctification through her life. I don't think I'm saying such great words, but for me Mioara is a saint, and others were sanctified through her, too.

EPILOGUE

3.
"The Testimony of a Shared Love"
*An Interview with Fr. Georgian Păunoiu,
St. Catherine Chapel of the Orthodox Theological Faculty,
Bucharest*

Father, when and how did you meet Mioara?

I met her a year ago, when I learned about her illness and suffering. My wife, Magda, was the first to find out about Mioara's trial, and from there on we got closer and closer — trying to know her family better, to be together with them. Actually, reflecting on the past, I realized we didn't give much of a revelation or help to Mioara, but rather Mioara gave us help in understanding our relationships with others, in our family, our bond with the children, our responsibility towards each other in the family. We didn't realize all these things from the beginning; they appeared later. Back then, things were all rolled up together in an avalanche, with her hospitalization, trying to be alongside Viorel and the children.... Thus, slowly, slowly, our souls became close.

What impressed you the most about Mioara?

The most beautiful thing was that, when you met her, even from the first encounter, she would be so warm and so natural, as if you had known each other for years. I see this as her special and rare gift — welcoming people into her soul, opening her heart to them. She would embrace you; there was no distance there, there was not the calculation that a person usually makes: "Wait a minute, we're just seeing each other for the first time...." Viorel and the children were the same. Anyway, this is how I always felt them: like one breath. That is to say, when they were all together in one place, they were one: the parents and the children.

How was the atmosphere at the wake and at the funeral? How did you sense the people?

I saw the people come to the two days of the wake as to a pilgrimage. Tens and hundreds of people—very close friends and those who knew her less. They came to pray for Mioara, to bid her farewell, and to entrust her to God the Bridegroom and to His love. During those days I felt great hope in the souls of the people I saw at Mioara's coffin. I saw pain, but also an enormous and unshakable faith that Mioara had left in peace and that, through God's work and mercy, she had prepared herself to meet Him—that she had prepared for her departure, and met Christ.

Many of those who went to bid her farewell said that they felt peace and joy in their souls. How can these states be explained?

I think about all those who read Mioara's book. I believe there is no one who did not shed tears, even sob, in reading the book, experiencing together with her the entire series of circumstances, of memories. You see, I believe God gave Mioara an extraordinary affective memory, which she had her entire life.

The people who came and wept at her coffin on the day of her funeral could not but observe her luminous face, full of peace, which, without any exaggeration or conjecture, expressed spiritual reconciliation, revealed detachment, and seemed to say farewell through the serenity and light that came from it. There are funerals where the atmosphere is quite oppressive, but nothing like that was felt at Mioara's funeral. On the contrary.

Did you sense that Christ was present in the midst of those escorting her?

Yes, indeed, Christ was present then, as He was before, accompanying Mioara all those years — six years of true martyrdom, of her battle with illness, of her hope, of hope conveyed to others, also. How wonderful it is not to be stuck in your suffering, not to pity yourself and only expect consolation, but on the contrary, to feel yourself called by God to strengthen others — you, the sick one.

This comes from a tremendous interior strength, and from a belief in, and consciousness of, the other person. The fact that Mioara would feel the other person very acutely was definitely one of her virtues and spiritual gifts. She would be able to touch such a profound chord of the other's soul that this motivated the person, charged him with trust, helped him look forward and not give in — and this in just a few words. Her might was not in words — she would often get very emotional, even flustered — but in the [spiritual] state she would convey.

Father, how could we, helpless and weak people of today, follow Mioara in virtue?

I believe that Mioara's testimony is that of a shared love. It is a stubbornness, if you will, to believe, to confess God's love, which is revealed most convincingly and powerfully through people. Mioara confessed this numerous times in her book, in her words, and in everything that she shared with others through her spiritual state.

4.
Message of Condolence from His Holiness Daniel, Patriarch of Romania

Read at the Funeral Service of Mioara Grigore, Saints George and Demetrios Parish of Călăgăău, Tărtășești, Dâmbovița County, Wednesday, March 4, 2015[6]

WITH PROFOUND Christian sorrow we received the news of the passing from this life, after arduous suffering, of Mrs. Mioara Grigore, religion teacher, devout wife, mother of five children, and pious daughter of our Church.

Six years ago, at the age of forty-four, Mrs. Mioara Grigore was diagnosed with (breast) cancer. Then the doctors did not give her much chance of survival, but she did not lose her faith and hope in God, the Holy Giver of Life, Whom she begged to give her a few more days for the sake of her children. The love, prayers, and support of her children, husband, and friends eased her journey through difficult times of suffering.

In the wake of her experience of a terrible disease, Mioara Grigore wrote the book *Cancer, My Love*. In it, she spoke about her suffering, which she lived through with much hope and unwavering faith, about human life and health as gifts of God, and about the importance of love in the family, especially, when there are many trials and adversities. Loved by her family and those around her, Mioara Grigore represents for

---

[6] Following the funeral Mioara was buried in the cemetery of Tărtășești, near her home.

EPILOGUE

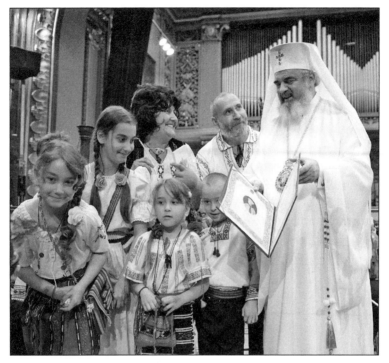

Patriarch Daniel presenting the Honorary Diploma "Maria Brâncoveanu" to Mioara on the occasion of the concert "Joy of the Resurrection" at the Romanian Athenaeum in Bucharest, May 19, 2014.

those who knew and loved her the model of a Christian wife and mother, who devoted her entire life to her family, with much love and joy, virtues that she wished to share with others through writing.

Last year, in 2014, when the three hundredth anniversary of the Brâncovenian Martyrs was commemorated in the Romanian Patriarchate, we gave Mrs. Mioara Grigore the "Maria Brâncoveanu" honorary diploma as a sign of our esteem for her devotion as a Christian mother. On this occasion we saw her husband and five children—Maria, Anthony, Nektarios, Macrina, and Justina—whom she raised with great love and sacrifice....

We pray that our merciful God will give rest to the soul of His handmaiden Mioara together with the righteous in the Heavenly Kingdom. May all those mourning be strengthened in the hope of the General Resurrection and in the communion and merciful love of our Savior Jesus Christ, the Crucified and Risen One.

May her memory be eternal!

His Holiness Daniel,
Patriarch of Romania

Appendix 1

"Sacrificing Oneself for Another Is an Overwhelming Miracle"

Interviews with Mioara and Viorel in 2013

Editor's Note: The following interviews were conducted by Raluca Tănăseanu and published in *Familia Ortodoxă* [The Orthodox Family] in February and March of 2013,[7] over a year before the publication of *Cancer, My Love*. The first interview (Part 1) is with Mioara, and the second (Part 2) is with both her and Viorel.

These interviews—as also the ones presented in Appendices 2 and 3—have been condensed. In several places we have made abridgements in order to avoid repeating what has been written elsewhere in the book. At the same time, we have retained some overlap, especially in places where the interviews offer new insights not found in Mioara's book.

A Story about Love Conquering Death
Part 1

Cancer. Five children. One of them with Down syndrome.

---

[7] *Familia Ortodoxă*, nos. 49 and 50.

CANCER, MY LOVE

Infinite love. This in just a few words is the portrait of a woman I have loved from the first time I met her. Without further introduction we invite you to meet her, too.

MIOARA, *you sent us an essay entitled "Heroes and Superheroes" for a writing contest organized by our magazine. In it, you wrote about the love between you and your husband. Your words touched us deeply. Tell us, how did it all begin?*

Both my husband and I had an unnaturally long childhood. Each of us lived with our mothers well into our thirties. When I met him I had just graduated with my Theology degree, and I found a teaching job in a high school. On the first day of the school year I was welcomed by my new students with bunches of flowers. I was trying to carry them all in my arms when suddenly I stumbled on my skirt and fell down the stairs. I literally landed on my future husband, who was also a teacher in that high school. I was very embarrassed by my own clumsiness. I asked him, "Are you hurt, Professor?" He said to me, "No, but I'm happy we met like this."...

When did you find God in your life?

Unfortunately, it was quite late in my life. It happened through my brother when I was around thirty. I had spent my life until then studying. My brother took me with him to Fr. Arsenie Papacioc. I still remember the first question Fr. Arsenie asked me then: "If you were to die today in an accident, how would you present yourself before God?" I had no answer to that. When I went out from that first Confession it started to rain. It was a beautiful summer rain. And that cool rain after my Confession with Fr. Arsenie made me feel literally "washed" and renewed. I felt as if I had been born again, as if a new life had been given to me....

Before studying theology you had been an actress. What was the transition from acting to theology like?

I don't really want to talk now about that period of my life. I feel they were wasted years. My life was more or less a tragedy then. I didn't need to act it—I was already living it. In those years my father was very sick. I was suffering terribly. I was fighting for his life. I only managed to play one role before deciding to study theology. My decision came after I made a bet with my brother that I could do it. He said I wouldn't be able to start all over again with studying, taking exams, and so on. His reaction motivated me to prove him wrong. I had a scholarship for the entire four years of my studies.

I was relying on my powerful memory, and I wasn't living what I was learning. I was missing the very spirit of theology. But I had professors who were a great influence on me. Gradually I learned to look at people with more love. I started to attend every Holy Liturgy. During my studies I met wonderful people. When I was thirty-three I thought to myself that, since I still wasn't married, I would probably become a nun. For about two years I kept thinking about St. Anthony the Great. I thought no man could reach even a quarter of his holiness, and I compared other men with him, so I found no motivation to marry. But, although I thought I'd be a nun, my spiritual father told me to stay home and take care of my sick mother after my father had passed away.

According to the doctors, my mother was supposed to

have died thirty years ago, but she confounded their prognosis and she is alive to this day, glory to God! She's a typical, old-fashioned peasant woman, very strong....

Do you think that having cancer made the love between you and your husband stronger?

It really did. Because I was able to discover his huge capacity of self-sacrifice and patience. In the hospital I met women who were crying because their husbands had left them. Maybe the husbands weren't very guilty in the sense that they weren't mature; they couldn't carry the cross of being with a wife who, sooner or later, would die. But here were deserted women, and I couldn't understand—if there was love once, where could that love suddenly disappear to, when the wife needs help more than ever?

That's how I saw my husband in a new light. I was overwhelmed by his patience, his power to believe in my healing, his determination that I still have to live for our children.

There were times when I had to take twenty different pills a day. I was somehow stuck in a boundless sadness, but he would remember to give me each pill on time, every two or three hours. He squeezed mountains of oranges for three years because I was vomiting from the chemotherapy....

For how long have you had cancer?

It started five years ago, while I was breastfeeding my youngest, Justina. A nodule appeared, and it hurt.... Eventually, my husband took me to Bucharest for tests, and they did a biopsy. We were told it was cancer, and moreover that it was very advanced. We were shocked, especially as I had been breastfeeding for years. We started to fight with it. Actually, my husband did most of the fighting for me. Sometimes in the hospital hallways I was worried he would pass out. We were just holding onto each other.

That's how I discovered the sacrificial aspect of love—the sacrifice of one for the other. I probably wouldn't have known such a thing as this—the overwhelming miracle of sacrificing oneself for another—if I hadn't had cancer.... I can only weep and thank God for giving me this disease.

There were times when we slept in separate rooms. I was embarrassed to sleep in the same bed with him because I thought I smelled of poison from all the treatments. But even from the other room he would sense when I was feeling sick, when I couldn't sleep, and he would come without me calling him and bring me a glass of freshly squeezed orange juice. To me those glasses of freshly squeezed orange juice are absolute love.

This January we celebrated twelve years of marriage. In these twelve years he's always called me "my love."... He knows how to keep fresh the feeling of the beginning of our love. He would drive me to the hospital and then wait for six hours until I finished my treatment. I would watch him through the window. He looked cold and hungry and full of worries, but even so I would feel butterflies in my stomach, and when he came in, instinctively I would arrange my wig. He would smile at me and embrace me, and his love would make me feel like a teenager. Through him I understood that the most important quality in a man is patience. I never had patience myself.

Beside your family, who supports you in this difficult trial?

Only recently did I understand why I need to thank God for this trial—because through it I met the most wonderful people in the world. Cancer brought into my life people whose hands I could kiss day and night, and about whom I could speak for days and nights, if I had the opportunity. People with extraordinary dedication to me—a stranger, basically. People who became so involved in my life, both financially—with money for various treatments—and spiritually, with their prayers. I'm so sorry they won't allow me to name them. But my children include a long list of benefactors in their prayers, and an evening doesn't pass without saying their names. One night, one of the children, Anthony, couldn't sleep because he had forgotten to pray for a certain gentleman. For me, for my husband and our children, these people are not only heroes, they're saints, and words fail me when I try to thank them. But five little children remember them in their innocent prayers.

Has all this suffering you've been through brought you closer to God?

Certainly. But this closeness has been mixed with a kind of desperation. I remember how one day, being unable to cry in front of my children, I went to the back of the garden and I cried and cried like never before in forty-five years. It was uncontrollable. It was a relief to be able to cry like that. And one of my girls, Macrina, heard me and came from behind me, wiped my tears with her little hands and told me with simplicity, "Don't cry, Mommy! Two breasts was in your way. They was too many. They was too heavy. One's better." And then I stopped crying. My children have such a pure way of looking at things. They're so innocent. I'll never be able to see the world as they do....

All these little gestures of my children overwhelm me. Obviously, I have a desperation that I shouldn't have, being a teacher of religion—in the sense that I haven't succeeded in entrusting everything to God. I know that, after my death, God won't leave all five children ... but they're so small, and Nektarios needs special care. When your lungs are full of cancer, you can't think about the distant future.

What hurts you the most, as you bear this cross?

Once I went to see my spiritual father, and there up in the mountains, in his small cell, he asked me, "What hurts you the most, Mioara?" There was so much gentleness in his voice that I felt it took away all the pain in the world. I showed him the window, and I said, "That hurts me the most, Father!" There, outside the window, were my husband with two of our children in his arms and three beside him. My spiritual father then told me something so simple, yet so deep and comforting, that for a while afterwards my inner turmoil disappeared. He said to me, "If you love your husband and children so much, won't God love them more? Won't He take care of them more [than you will]?" I left as if on wings.

I'm sorry that I've had and still have this heavy sin on my soul: that I've loved my children more than God. That's why I suffer. Nevertheless, I have hope that I'll yet understand and give myself over, once and for all, to the will of God. I still ache for them, like any mother, but if I were stronger and more anchored in faith, I think I wouldn't suffer so much.

Part 2

Mioara, is it difficult to raise five children in today's world?

MIOARA: I was on maternity leave for nine years in a row because the children came one after another. When I went back to work after nine years, the school inspector didn't believe me when I said I had five children and cancer. So the next day I went with all five children to his office. He was stunned. He asked me if they were really my children and not my grandchildren. Many people who meet us think they are our grandchildren because we got married and had them late.

These wonderful children have brought us closer to God. Especially Nektarios. My husband should tell you about everything this child brought into our lives.

VIOREL: Together with Nektarios many miracles came into our lives. Actually, ever since we met, our lives have been filled with miracles. I remember when we first went to Fr. Adrian Fageteanu—it was then I started to understand what the Orthodox Faith means. I was very far away from it. I used to think I was the center of the universe. The smartest, the best. You know, you can't come to know God at student parties. You meet Him in despair, in suffering. I had the great opportunity of meeting my wife. Through her I found God. Through her I found a spiritual father. I had always been looking for the truth, for the meaning of all this, and had always felt that something was missing. I used to read a lot of philosophy, but I couldn't find myself in it. I had, and still have, a passion for mathematics. I think there's a subtle connection between mathematics and God—everything is precision.

APPENDIX I

What was your outlook on life before finding God?

Life was purely material, a differential equation with some solutions. I was a misogynist. I had no wish to get married. I was a loner.

My mother, God rest her soul, used to go to church. I'd take her by car every Sunday, but I'd never go into the church myself; I'd wait outside. Still, I used to reflect: Why is she going? She used to fast, but she would cook separately for me and my father. She never asked us to fast, but she kept a very strict fast. She was so delicate. God is delicate—He never imposes anything on us.

After my father passed away, I was left with a big plot of land. Around that time we had a big drought, and I started to be angry with God. So much so that even I realized I wasn't sane anymore. It was then that I met this wonderful wife of mine, and she saved me....

What drew you to her?

Her determination to drag me towards God. I said to myself, "This woman wants to make something out of my life." That pilgrimage to St. Parasceva was a miracle in my life. I can't even find the right words to describe it. I was an atheist when I went, and when I came back I would have jumped to fight if someone told me there was no God. That was the beginning of my conversion to faith, but I feel it's a lifelong process. Before, I used to feel an emptiness inside. I couldn't carry on living like that. In all of us there's a judge: our conscience. It works and works even if we ignore it, and then there comes a moment when you can't keep ignoring it and you start asking yourself some questions, you start looking within yourself.

Going back to Nektarios: have you ever blamed God for giving you this cross of having a child with Down syndrome?

Yes. At some point, in my stupidity and lack of faith, I started to blame God, to fall into despondency: "Why, God, did you give me this cross? Why to me? Don't you see I do this and that, I go to church ..." In those moments the interior struggles are very hard. Only a good spiritual father can guide you in how to fight these thoughts that are constantly attacking you. I realized that it all came from my pride, that the beast in me hadn't died, and that Nektarios had, in fact, given us many miracles.

As soon as he came into our lives, God sent wonderful people our way. Former colleagues from the university called and asked if they could help. People who don't necessarily go to church but even so have a great spirit of sacrifice; people who are ready to help. To me this was extraordinary. Maybe if it wasn't for Nektarios I wouldn't have been in touch with these people. This in itself was a miracle.

Once I went to Frasinei Monastery, the "Romanian Athos." That monastery is my "spiritual school." Nektarios was close to death at the time. He had a congenital malformation in his heart, and was scheduled for surgery. My wife was praying to St. Nektarios at home. I went to Frasinei and asked a father there, "Father, what am I to do? I'm through ..." Of course, I was thinking in a worldly way. The father told me to glorify God, because if Nektarios were to die we would have an angel praying for us in heaven. His words brought be back to my senses. I realized what a huge distance there is between true faith—real monastic faith—and a worldly, comfortable faith.

APPENDIX I

When I went back home, I was so relieved. I understood that, whatever happened, it was God's will. Nektarios was cured miraculously, without any surgery, and shortly afterwards we found out that my wife was expecting our fourth child. Doubts crept in again.... What should we do? After having a child with Down syndrome we were apprehensive about having another child. Even our doctor, who was a very faithful and dedicated woman, wasn't encouraging us to go ahead with such a risky pregnancy. As we were walking around the hospital yard, both of us feeling numb, in a state of futility, I suddenly had a thought: "Mioara, God sees how stupid and weak we are. He can't give us another child with a handicap!" I really felt very stupid.

And, glory to God, we had a healthy child. That decision was very dramatic and important. A great turning point in our lives. We could have become criminals if we had given in to fear.

MIOARA: Several doctors told us then that Macrina would be a vegetable. And when she was born she was 5.2 kilos [11.4 lbs.]. We both fought hard, she and I, when she came into the world. We almost died. I delivered her without a C-section, and it felt like my eyes almost popped out due to the pain of delivering such a huge baby. But she was very healthy.

The doctors couldn't believe their eyes. Someone from a local newspaper came to interview me, the woman who delivered a huge baby without a C-section. How could I do it? Nobody knew in advance how big the baby actually was. When I was seven months pregnant they told me she was too small, so I started eating and eating, and she grew and grew. In two months she reached that amazing weight.

VIOREL: Our doctor was in trouble after this delivery. She was fired because the hospital management considered there had been a high risk of mortality. For the hospital management we were numbers, statistics. This is the system. If you're over forty there's a high risk when you give birth, in any case. They reproached our doctor for allowing my wife to give birth without a C-section. But this doctor fought a lot for us, and she was a good match for my wife, who's also a fighter. That's the great rift between the world of those who only know science and the world of God's wonders.

Let's go back to Nektarios. How do you communicate with him?

MIOARA: With difficulty. Recently he started to talk, mainly due to his brothers and sisters, who always talk to him. I remember the first time he ever said something. I was in the kitchen talking with my husband, "Daddy," I said, "I don't think our baby will ever talk." Then, not knowing where Nektarios was in the house, I said to Viorel, "Look around, where is Nektarios now?"

The next moment Nektarios, from out of the hallway, said, "Here I am."

That was his first sentence. We celebrated all day. I realized it was yet another miracle, and acknowledged that we don't have trust and patience.

At school they make fun of him sometimes. They call him "dummy." Macrina comes home crying every time her little brother gets bullied. All four children protect him and fight for him.

APPENDIX I

Nektarios can be very stubborn sometimes. If you tell him not to do something, he will surely do it a thousand times. He has a stubbornness that forces you to learn patience.

For a year now, I can't stay inside the church with him during the services because he keeps saying in a loud voice, "Amen. Amen. Lord, Lord." He doesn't stop. He says he's "serving," too. I go out with him, we walk around the church. He's starting to realize that he's different, that he can't talk like the other children can, and he becomes angry and agitated, but then he calms down. Lately I've noticed a very good development in him, and we thank God for that.

When I reprimand him, he comes and puts his arms around my neck and says to us, "Mommy, I lobe you! Daddy, I lobe you very much!" Whenever I discipline him, not with anger but with the wish to teach him, he cries and then comes to me and hugs and kisses me. By doing so, he's teaching me. He's so simple. He's like a little saint. Maybe it sounds over the top to say so, but the saints always reacted to rebukes with love—and Nektarios does exactly the same. He doesn't have anything evil in him, any desire for revenge.

Sometimes his brothers and sisters leave him out, because he doesn't vibrate on the same wavelength as they do. If his own siblings isolate him sometimes, society will isolate him for sure. He'll inevitably be marginalized, bullied. This is a cross he began to carry from birth. A very difficult cross. But also a great opportunity for salvation.

Mioara, what makes you happy?

Everything in my life, with very few exceptions, makes me happy. The fact that both my husband and I have a spiritual father who keeps us in his heart, takes care of our souls, and carries our cross with us. The fact that we have five children who are wise and constantly teach us amazing life lessons. The fact that we've met wonderful people who overwhelm us with their spirit of sacrifice.... And I still have time to learn to be happy. I hope I won't die before I learn to enjoy this battle with cancer. If I had the capacity to fully experience the joy and honor that God has given me along with this disease, if I had the power to rejoice in this sadness, then I'd be truly happy.

Do you think that relationships between people have deteriorated in recent years?

In some ways. On the one hand, when I went back to work at the high school where I had been a teacher, my colleagues were amazing. I discovered these wonderful women, who have difficult lives, with long, tiring commutes to school, women who leave home at 4 a.m. to get to work. Maybe they don't go to church every Sunday, but they have the capacity to understand the suffering of others, to build relationships of love and respect. I realized people can go on if they at least have this spark of compassion and understanding of others.

On the other hand, the students were different from nine years ago. I was shocked. Before, they used to have a sense of shame, of respect towards their teachers. When I went back to teaching after nine years, I found some angry kids, confused, loud, and without any values to guide their lives. But seeing me as I was—bald, yellow, running to the bathroom to throw up at every break—they changed, and in the end they gave me great strength to carry on!

APPENDIX I

Every time I would come to class they would ask me to tell them more about the lives of saints. Every day they would tell me I was beautiful. And I was looking awful. This bunch of angry and confused kids gave me strength to keep fighting. I realized then that even when they were swearing, even when they were fighting, even when they were vulgar, they still had some innocence, they still had the image of God in them.

Why do think the youth have changed?

They've become estranged from their own selves. They can't find peace in anything. In the beginning I was more judgmental towards them. I was thinking they could at least be quiet during class. They were constantly talking, they couldn't be still at their desks, they were in a continuous agitation. But when I got to know them better, I realized that their home environments were terrible: parents with large debts, facing hardship, laboring in the fields. The parents themselves had behavioral and social problems.

Still, what drew them to your classes?

I wasn't so much following a curriculum, but rather talking to them about God's immense love. I was telling them about the lives of saints, and encouraging them to apply in their own lives what they heard in class, to improve themselves. They became quiet and attentive because I was talking to them about their issues. Some had tears in their eyes, and they would come to me after class and tell me, "You know, I have this problem ..."

This closeness brought me so much joy. I was humbled and honored whenever they shared a secret of their soul with me. More than air to breathe, they needed someone to talk to, someone who cared. And they were giving me so much strength to fight. I was poisoned, bald, but they were telling me how beautiful I was to them.

I was just telling them stories. Young people of seventeen and eighteen, who were still mad about stories! Perhaps they enjoyed going back to their childhood, to a time less threatening, less vulgar, less complicated.

Mioara, what would you say to others who have heavy crosses to bear like yourself?

Not to fall into despondency as I did. And I regret it so much. I feel ashamed, because there was a time when I had in my soul a sadness bordering on despair. I hope I never get to that point again. I'm ashamed for what I felt then. I would tell anyone not to fall into despondency, because when they least expect it a miracle will come! I didn't hope or expect a miracle, and yet so many miracles have happened. Perhaps they came for my children. The very fact that I'm alive now is a miracle.

I feel I haven't deserved so many miracles, and still they've come into my life. Each time I was in labor and it was taking forever, I would send my husband to the wonderworking icon of the Theotokos at Ghighiu Monastery. He would get there, and I would deliver in a few minutes after ten to twenty hours of labor.

Then, when I had cancer, I would go to the icon and ask her, "Panagia, I beg you, one more year, that's all I ask. I want Justina to be five. She's too small now to lose her mommy. She still can't fall asleep unless I'm there and she feels my cheeks between her palms." I was asking Panagia in my despair, "What stepmother would bear to have this girl smother her at night with her hands on her cheeks in this impossible heat?" (It was summer then, and it was very hot, even at night). "Who's going to sit there, with her cheeks being held in the hands of my little girl?" So I asked Panagia for a year. And a year passed, and I lived. Then I went to our spiritual father and told him. "Father, I'm ashamed to ask for another year. I feel so cowardly and pathetic.... What can I say?" He smiled and said, "Then let's pray that you can go into overtime."

Again he gave me strength. And I've been praying, together with my children and with many extraordinary people, for God to give me some more "overtime."

Appendix 2

"I Would Die from the Happiness of Being Able to Live!"

An Interview with Mioara and Viorel in 2014

EDITOR'S NOTE: The following interview was conducted by Raluca Tănăseanu and published in *Familia Ortodoxă* [The Orthodox Family], May 2014 (no. 64) pp. 31–37, shortly after the publication of the Romanian edition of *Cancer, My Love*.

BELOVED MIOARA, a year ago we interviewed you about your illness and five children. Our readers are asking us: what have you been doing since then?

MIOARA: I experienced the miracle of meeting some saints. I hope I won't shock you with this word, but I've come to understand that there are saints among us. These people have prolonged my life through their love. And so, I live in almost cosmic wonder—how is it that I haven't died yet? According to oncology, the cancer scattered in my lungs and liver should have taken over, devastating me completely. However, it seems that the love of these people has kept my metastases stagnant, and, moreover, these people have taken all the "bullets" of my pain. I believe the miracle God gave me of encountering them has greatly superseded the miracle of physical healing. I couldn't ask God for bodily healing anymore, as long as He has given me this overwhelming wonder of feeling the love of these people.

Love conquers all ...

Yes, indeed. I didn't believe it was possible, as I didn't believe it was possible to feel joy in suffering. And these are not just big words. I wouldn't want to seem hypocritical: I would give anything to be able to raise my children, to be able to be by their side, knowing, first of all, how much we love each other — like mad fools — and, secondly, how much they need their mommy — and I would die from the happiness of being able to live! But I've come to realize that much more vital than getting rid of cancer is this miracle: changing your thoughts, soul, heart, and being filled with love, seeing how much love God has put in a man when he sacrifices himself for his neighbor. And I experienced this miracle of feeling the sacrifice of others for me. The tears that inundate my heart and soul are most often precisely tears of utter gratitude to God for sending these saints into my life.

You wrote a book, recently released: Cancer, My Love. *Have you attained to loving cancer?*

Truly, it was a shocking title for many people, even for me, but it's very true. I kept thinking, night after night: what can I give these people who've done so much for me and my little ones? Being in a meager financial situation, and spiritually even more destitute, I felt so poor, and I didn't know what to give them.... And then I realized I could still give them

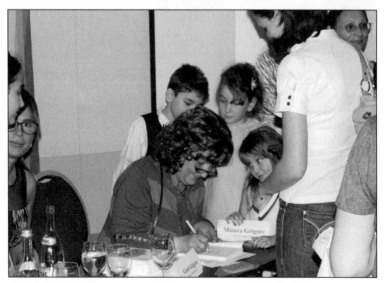

Presentation and book signing with the release of the Romanian edition of *Cancer, My Love,* March 21, 2014, Bucharest. *At right:* poster showing the Romanian cover design.

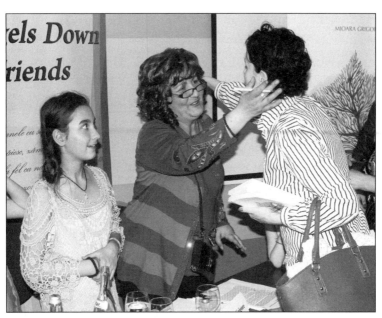

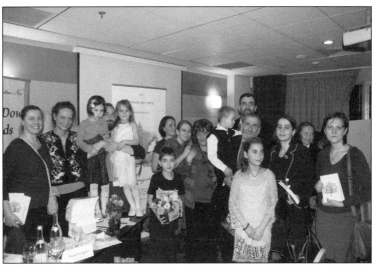

something through my children, praying for all these heroes we had—since in the meantime they had become our heroes! And as I continued reflecting on this in the desperate moments when they sustained me with their love, I understood that if I hadn't had this honorable illness—this cancer, which is often a nightmare!—I wouldn't have known the miracle of feeling their love.

How did the illness evolve during the past year?

This past year the metastases invaded the lung, and from the lung the cancer spread to the liver.... But I'm so glad it hasn't gone to the brain (which was because, as my husband well said, "My love, why would it go to the head, since you have nothing there?") This has encouraged me tremendously! It seems it hasn't spread to the bones, either. This is contrary to the [more common] pattern: from the lungs to the brain, from the brain to the bones, from the bones to the liver. But one thing is certain: it was impossible for it to enter my heart. Since I have so many loved ones there, there was no room for this cancer!

You spoke earlier about the spirit of sacrifice that gave you strength to go on. And yet, it's not every day that we find people who are able to sacrifice themselves for their neighbor. What makes people sacrifice what's theirs: their time, comfort, money, well-being, and ease?

I don't know, because this amazes me greatly and I'm completely overwhelmed, from head to toe: what made them sacrifice their time for me, for my family? What made them call me at night and ask me, "Are you hurting badly?" What made them buy food and clothing for the children? What made

APPENDIX 2

them embrace me every Sunday and tell me, "Although you don't believe you're going to live, we firmly believe!" The fact that they strongly believed in my place reveals precisely an element of godlikeness in them.

How meaningful is an outstretched hand for a suffering person?

Ah, how can I tell you? It's everything! It's life! It's God, it's love.... One night, unable to bear the pain in my bones, I called a friend and asked him, "Do you think I'll be able to endure the great pains that are cropping up?"—those pains that make you pray that God will take you sooner because you can't bear them anymore, those pains that make your brain explode in your head and your heart in your chest.... And I asked him then, "Do you think I'll be able to bear them?" He told me, "The great pains have already passed. Now the joys will come!" And all of a sudden he swept everything away.

Similarly, one night I bothered another friend. I called her and said, "What can I do? Because of the pain, I'm swinging myself in the armchair like a child." She said, "Mioriţule, I'm coming now to see you! What should I give you? What should I bring you?" She would buy me pills, and engulf me with inconceivable love. And so many, so many proofs of love.... A hand outstretched toward a suffering person is everything! I'm honestly telling you, it prolongs life.

Viorel, we were all surprised by your love for your wife, so movingly presented in the book. What makes the love between spouses remain as in the beginning, especially when one of them goes through difficult moments?

VIOREL: Well, first and foremost, this love is not a term taken out of the dictionary or found only in love poems, praised by art or literary critics—rather, it's a living word that comes from God.... We can't forget that the family is a mystery, marriage is a mystery, through which the grace of God ennobles and gives continuity to the small offerings of human beings on the path to salvation. The Christian family should be a pillar—a pillar of salvation. Salvation is said to be personal, but helping your neighbor starts from the fundamental cell, from the family. You can't say: "Now, I'm ready to help my 'neighbor' from Iași, from Târgoviște, from Constanța,"[8] while you're not helping your neighbor—or your close-neighbor, as I would refer to a family member. What can we say about love for God.... If there's no love for our neighbor, our love for God exists only in theological textbooks (cf. 1 John 4:20–21)!

Mioara, in the book you told us that you had moments of falling, when you felt you couldn't continue the battle. Where did you find strength to arise and continue?

MIOARA: To begin with, I looked into the eyes of our little ones, who would implore me to get out of bed, and beg me to stop crying. Maria, our oldest child, told me in a serious and sufficiently drastic tone, "Get up, dear, because you can't afford the luxury of depression now, when you have five children to raise, and an eighty-two-year-old paralyzed mother! Leave depression for later on!" What else could I do? And my husband would come and say, "My love, you're not allowed, you can't desert ... What are you doing to us?" I couldn't look back anymore. I had to stand there, up in front, and—whether

---

[8] Cities in different parts of Romania.

APPENDIX 2

I was able to resist or not — at least I had to try to be amazing and resist!

You've spent a lot of time in hospitals. What has impressed you the most about the cancer patients you've encountered?

The youth. The youth impressed me terribly, and I felt like a rag in their presence. They had a freedom, a strength, a steadfastness of soul! The acceptance of lambs, as the Savior says; they were like lambs. They didn't revolt, didn't fight with anyone, and also didn't resign themselves. They accepted suffering and death so beautifully! They weren't like us, the others, over forty years old — scrambling for every moment and willing to give anything to prolong our lives. For them everything was so smooth, and they were so much at peace with death that you'd think they had come straight out of the *Paterikon*.

VIOREL: I was deeply moved by the sincerity of the people we met who were suffering. It's a genuine sincerity, because people don't wear any masks at such times. Well, some might say, "They must be frightened people!" They're not frightened; they're people who've overcome their condition and are asking themselves existential questions — not about the verb "to have," but about the verb "to be"! And they go to the hospital as regular people, not separated by any demarcations: social, spiritual, financial, or whatever. What impressed me profoundly is that most of them, young and old, asked for God's help with extraordinary power, either openly or in private.

I would probably call this title, *Cancer, My Love,* a "mutagenic title," in the sense that it's a title that changes a paradigm. It brings about a paradigm mutation because the word "cancer" is associated with illness, despair, lamentation, and even with suicide, which leads to the loss of the soul—while for Mioara the title seeks to completely change this unpleasant facade. [In the book] cancer is shown to be a path to better self-knowledge and to victory—victory over death. It seems like a paradox, but there has to be a paradigm change; otherwise, you won't be able to live with this axe—cancer—hanging over your head.

Mioara, what would you recommend to those suffering from incurable illnesses? How can they escape dark thoughts that torment them?

MIOARA: It's not easy at all; the battle is terribly difficult. I know that, especially during long winter nights, when the pain seized me, it was very difficult to think, "It will be okay," or, "God won't leave me." At such moments, when my brain seemed to explode from so much pain, it was hard to find the strength ... but not impossible. I anchored myself, with my whole being, in the Mother of God, who, having the heart of a mother, knew the pain in my heart.

I was almost shocked by the help I felt so vividly from the Mother of God a month ago, when the doctors asked to do a MRI to see if the cancer had spread to my brain. I didn't know [in advance] how this brain MRI was to be done. At one point they placed me in a tube with some earphones, and they put on some noises that were so intense that I felt my brain would explode. My heart started racing; it was beating so hard that it seemed to ascend into my throat, while my tongue was descending. They had given me a little pump to squeeze if I felt sick, so the doctor would know and come to interrupt the entire procedure. But I wasn't able to squeeze the pump and, when I felt my tongue descending and my heart exploding in my chest, I cried to the Mother of God with all my being.

There were, I think, a few dozen extremely heavy, dire seconds, in which I concretely felt the quiver of death in my entire being. But I felt the help of the Mother of God so vividly that, at some point, I felt two hands, so soft and warm, going into my mouth and taking my tongue out of my throat slowly, slowly.... And then my heart calmed down little by little. So did my brain, although those infernal noises continued. Slowly, slowly she brought me back to life, and I got over it.

Therefore, I say: to whom are you going to cry out in those difficult moments, if not to the good God and His Mother? Since that incident I weep when I reflect on how I called out to the Mother of God just a little, and she didn't desert me. It was overwhelming!

Your book is a true public confession, in which you reveal your weaknesses, fears, renunciations, despair.... How can we gain the courage to discover our weaknesses and fight against them?

I don't know. I believe everyone will find the necessary courage at the appropriate moment. I admit that after the publication of this book I was almost ashamed to leave the house, because I knew it was a book about weakness, fear, cowardice—and I was wondering if someone would still love me, seeing me so weak and frail spiritually. But it was like a refreshing wind, like a rain after a drought!

After the publication of this book I received so many proofs of affection, understanding, compassion, and love that I rejoiced exceedingly. Nothing hurt me anymore. I believe my tumor markers dropped instantly when I saw how many people were and are beside me—reading this book and understanding perfectly what I wanted to say. I rejoiced that people with different educational backgrounds understood me—those who had finished graduate and postgraduate studies and those who hadn't finished middle school. It was a miracle for me that my weakness touched people's souls, and I was nourished by the courage they gave me. For example, someone told me, "After reading this book I want to die with you when you die." For me, that was something.... I don't know—divinely beautiful, and painfully beautiful. All these people gave me wings and strength.

Now, after going through so much suffering, what would you say that you appreciate the most in a person?

The spirit of sacrifice. This reveals the divine in a person. The spirit of sacrifice pushed to the annihilation of one's ego.... All these people I met providentially were not themselves anymore—they were me. The miracle I was given in meeting them made me experience (I didn't think it was possible!) the joy of feeling other people's joy. These people taught me how to rejoice in suffering, in the moments of pain, of despair. And the fact that I learned to rejoice in suffering gave me the strength to move forward. This is learned slowly, slowly, step by step—and if you've learned to acquire this joy you're able to overcome a whole lot. I need these people so much; I need their spirit of sacrifice tremendously. Without them I'm nothing....

Mioara, how can we see the beauty in every person? In the book you show us that we can learn something from any person. How can you benefit from the neighbor whom God, at some point, has placed next to you?

APPENDIX 2

At Fundeni Hospital I saw almost absolute beauty, divine beauty, when a young man, twenty-three years old, from Moldova, sat near my bed. He was a simple young man, who told me he only had ten years of schooling because his parents had no money to send him to school. He was thin, frail, with bandages on his head after an operation to remove a massive brain tumor, but he was so pure in spirit that you could sense the brightness, simplicity, and purity of his soul from afar.

So, he sat on his bed, and I saw that, having had a serious dose of chemotherapy, he had turned a bit green in the face. His heart stopped beating, and the nurses quickly gave him some shots to restart it. I asked him, "Did you eat anything this morning before leaving the house?" "No," he said, "because I stay with my brother and his wife in Bucharest, and they have a baby. They give me food, but I'm embarrassed to eat, for them to see me like this; I wouldn't want to disturb them… Anyway, I didn't escape my sister-in-law, and I took a sandwich with me. But as I was on the way to the hospital, a beggar, an old man, stretched his hand out to me so I could help him with something, since he hadn't eaten in two days … and what could I could do?"

And that young man gave him his only sandwich. He preferred to remain hungry, knowing that after the chemotherapy he could faint or even worse—he could have a heart attack—and he gave away his sandwich! I honestly tell you, his gesture seemed to me a sign of sanctity. I looked at him; I wanted to buy him something to eat, but he didn't accept my offer, saying, "I know you have little children.… No, I'll be all right. I'll go to my brother's house and eat." His soul was so simple and beautiful! Afterwards I couldn't resist—I went outside and wept with joy that God had put so much goodness in man!

If you were to encounter the Savior, what would you ask of Him?

Well, you know, as a mother, my heart aches for the children. I would only ask God to strengthen their souls so they won't be terribly sad when I'm gone, because they tell me every day, 'Mommy, you'll stay with us and we'll be together, right?' And Nektarios, our boy with Down syndrome, who is now nine years old, has learned to say a few phrases, and every night he just says, 'My Mommy, don't go-o, don't go-o!' If I go, if God allows this, I would ask of Him this: that all my five children would not be seized by sadness!

VIOREL: First of all, I would ask Him to leave the gate of heaven a bit open for my wife, and to bring an abundance of peace and enlightenment of mind to our family. To give Mioara some "extra time" in this transitory life, which is full of many blessings as well as temptations. And to continue to give the children the childhood they need....

Since we just celebrated Pascha, I would like to ask you: what do you think we have to do for the resurrection of our souls? I say this because, although our bodies may be healthy and strong, our souls are numb, if not dead.

MIOARA: Let's look a little in the direction of the other person, our neighbor, and discover in his eyes how much he needs us. We have an immense, imperious, total need for our neighbor's love! I once heard a Father say something colossal in a sermon: "Let us fall in love again with one another!" If we were to fall in love with each other again, we would truly feel the joy of living.

Many thanks for the interview! Christ Is Risen! And may we do an interview about your many grandchildren, years and years from now!

Oh, that seems so far away! I'm amazed and greatly rejoice when the sun rises and I'm still alive, when I'm still breathing—heavily, in all honesty, but still breathing—and when every night the little hands of our five children hug my back and caress my lungs, lungs full of metastases but also full of their love.... I believe that this is life: the privilege to rejoice in every moment with your loved ones, and in everything God has given you.

Appendix 3

"I'm Not Alone— I'm with Mioara"

Interviews with Viorel and Maria in 2016

Editor's Note: The following interview was conducted by Raluca Tănăseanu and published in *Familia Ortodoxă* [The Orthodox Family], March 2016 (no. 86) pp. 33–39, a year after Mioara's repose.

Viorel, it's been a year since Mioara passed away. How has this year been for your family?

Viorel: It's been a difficult year, of course. A year full of trials. The physical absence of their mother has been very hard for the children. In its place, however, we've felt Mioara's help from heaven, and so things have carried on naturally. The children, glory to God, passed through as well as possible this supreme trial of losing their mother and their primary mentor, who in our family was Mioara. In the process they've become more focused on family life, more determined to move forward. Their way of dealing with the new reality has helped me to become better, and to deal more diligently with the problems inherent in this separation.

I felt Mioara's help first of all in the fact that the children did not succumb to sadness. This, for me, is a miracle—only God could do that! Also, I felt her help in the great crowd of people who came to us with open arms, helping us financially, and especially spiritually. Through their prayers and the prayers of our spiritual father (Fr. Arsenie from Cornu), we came out of this stronger spiritually. Daily life is a struggle in today's secular, godless world. I had the great opportunity to live with a saint, and this to me is the greatest blessing.

Do you ask Mioara to help you as you would ask a saint?

Yes. I find it natural to do so because her life was not a normal life. The virtues she acquired can only be gained through a life of holiness.

Do you hear testimonies from people who say they also feel help?

Yes. Many ask me if I've had a dream about Mioara. I haven't. Perhaps she sees me as too stupid and doesn't want to trouble me. But there are others who've dreamed of her, even in some extraordinary circumstances. They see her happy, in a world without suffering, a world completely different from the one she left behind—because here on earth she tasted hell, so to speak. You can't taste heaven without going through a little hell, too.

What do people say to you about Mioara's book?

Mioara's book is a miracle. The reception has been overwhelming—from simple people to university professors, from lay people to monastics, from priests to senators, from bakers to school teachers. It's a book that brings a lot of comfort. Some say it should be read after the Bible—I think that's an exaggeration, but it's their opinion. It can, however, serve as a guidebook for the spiritual life of every person, for it reflects a life full of suffering and gives one a certain strength to continue one's own struggles.

Maria resembles her mother a lot. How is she? Is she a "miniature Mioara"?

Definitely. Beyond the physical resemblance she's very strong, very direct, very determined. She's mature beyond her years. She also took over in taking care of her sick grandmother, Mioara's mother, who has also passed away. All these experiences were a true school for her. Very few children today go through what she's gone through. I think all this has shaped her for life. Maria is not someone to sweat over small things. She never will be. The exams she takes at school are nothing compared to the life exams she's had to take.

Now she's my rock in the house. She helps with everything, from keeping things in order and cleaning to taking care of her younger siblings. She's a real professor in miniature. I'm happy to have such a support in her....

Do you consult with her when making important decisions for your family, like you used to consult with Mioara?

I include all the children in all the decisions we have to make for our family. I talk to each of them according to their age, but I involve them all. There have been plans that have been cancelled because they didn't agree with them. I always try to respect their point of view—unless it's something completely absurd, of course. But I consult with them

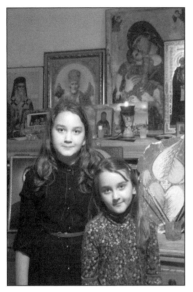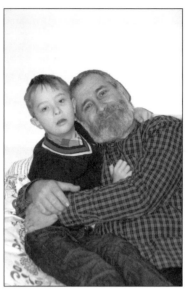

The Grigore family at their home, February 18, 2016.
Photos by Mircea Stanciu (Anca's husband).

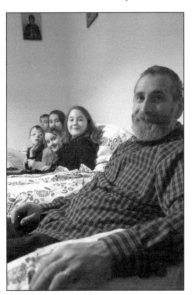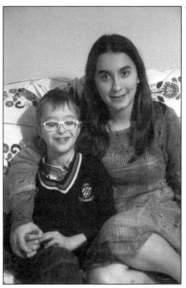

in all matters, and we try to stay united, as Mioara taught us.

Returning to Mioara: People's love helped her tremendously. I'm convinced that your loved ones surrounded you with love, as well. How important for you was the love of those around you?

It mattered immensely, because in such circumstances, if you're alone and not surrounded by friends, if you don't at least receive a comforting word or a hug, it's very difficult. We were accustomed to having a lot of friends, and Mioara was nourished through these people—and so was I. They supported me, encouraged me, joked with me, helped me with the children.... It was extremely important for me, and for the children, that we didn't find ourselves alone.

These people helped us with the installation of our heating system, with buying fuel, with groceries and clothing. We were surrounded with love all the time, not only from those close to us, but also from many people we never met, who gave us from the "widow's mite." This was profoundly moving.

Viorel, what have been the hardest moments this last year?

Hard moments occur all the time, but I try to overcome them. I always say to myself that nothing is harder than what Mioara went through. She went through a kind of martyrdom. Her pains were perhaps comparable to those endured in Communist prisons. I don't know if they were of the same intensity, but they weighed so heavily on the soul that, in experiencing only a tiny fraction of them, I felt I was being torn apart.

I try to understand this lesson that was given to us. I realize that, in God's providence, it happened for a purpose. I try to carry on living by remembering my wife's courage while dying.

I'm a simple student of a religion teacher who fought with death and conquered it.

What about the best moments?

The best moments were all the instances when I discovered something I didn't know about my wife. I found out about things she had done without my knowledge. People she had helped. Charity she had done. People I don't know come to me and tell me, "I knew your wife and she gave me this or that," or, "If I said she had a nice coat, she'd immediately take it off and give it to me. I was afraid to mention [I liked] anything else." These stories bring me joy and strengthen me.

I'm also happy when I meet her former students. There are some extraordinary people who have been following her advice, and I rejoice to see them doing well in life. They speak of her with great respect.

I'm happy that her book is alive and that it touches so many lives.

Lastly, I'm happy to see my children's motivation and determination to move forward in life....

Will there be a second book?

There will be a second volume. Mioara wrote two chapters. I'll try to put on paper most of [the rest of] what happened. It's very challenging for me to write. After all, it's a talent....

There will be a special chapter on her passing into the next life. I had the blessing to be beside her when she passed, and I'll try to depict the moment as it happened. There will also be a few chapters with more unusual stories, with all sorts of wondrous and unheard-of adventures we really experienced. I believe we won't write a very beautiful second volume, but we'll make a very useful one, as a continuation of the story Mioara began.

Nonetheless, you are a man raising five children alone. How does one of your days pass?

Well, I'm not alone—I'm with Mioara, and I have God's help. It's grievous if you're alone in the world. Only godless people are alone; it's really difficult to live like that.

The day begins at around 6 a.m., with an attempt to make breakfast, and with the awakening of Nektarios. Nektarios has good days, when he wants to go to school, and days that aren't so good, when he doesn't want to go to school; days when he says "yes," and then when we're about to leave he says "no," and we try a thousand times to convince him to go, and he goes between "yes" and "no." Then the children make up all kinds of scenarios, with incentives like "pizza," "little cars," "small trains," and so on, trying to convince him. In some cases we all fail, and I have to leave him at home because otherwise the others would miss school. This for me is the key moment of the morning, the "Nektarios moment," in which Nektarios decides whether or not he wants to go to school.

Then I drive the five children to school, the older ones to their school and then Nektarios to a special school. I drop off the older ones first, because Nektarios doesn't want to get out of the car until all the other children are out—otherwise he feels abandoned.

Then I come home and I chop some wood, make the fire,

and try to cook some food. I try to mail some books, to read two or three passages from a book, to say a "Lord, have mercy!" if I can. Afterwards, I go to pick Nektarios up at 2 p.m., since he finishes earlier than the others. Next, if Nektarios is hungry, I give him some soup. Then I pick up the other children from school. In the meantime I may have to go to a parent-teacher conference, but I'm grateful to the teachers for not calling me very often.

Then we get home, set the table, and have the evening meal. After this the problems arise: second-grade arithmetic problems, third-grade arithmetic, followed by eighth-grade problems with the theorem of the three perpendiculars and with calculating the volume of a closed surface, then Romanian syntax and morphology problems, then English-language questions: vocabulary, word order, and the usage of commas. Then second-grade problems concerning "apples," "pears," "grapes," and "Anna"—and finally we have some time for prayer before sleep.

Viorel, now you are a father and a mother for your children. What have been the most beautiful gestures through which they've shown their gratitude and love to you?

Just the fact that they're not sad, that they mimic their joy very well—because I feel it's a "worked on" joy; it's not a joy that comes as it is of itself, in full. It's a joy with a bit of "makeup," to make me rejoice in their joy. This is a gesture of utmost love, which I appreciate immensely. It's also a gesture of love that they try to be obedient to me, to confer with me. It's a gesture of love that they go to church and want to commune—this is a gesture of love towards God, first and foremost.

A simple gesture of love was the mere fact that, a few days ago, Macrina and Justina secluded themselves for about two hours and then put a sign with a heart on the kitchen door: "For Daddy." Approaching, I saw the kitchen very clean, organized, with the dishes clean and the floor mopped. It was a gesture that shocked me. That heart was bright red, very beautiful, with the inscription: "For Daddy." Well, for daddy this is a major gesture; there's no greater statement of love than this. It was extraordinary.

In your opinion, what was Mioara's greatest virtue?

Mioara's greatest virtue was her generosity and total self-sacrifice, giving herself completely for her neighbor, no matter if it was her husband, her children, or others she greatly loved.

Viorel, we thank you, and we pray that God will also give us a little bit of this love Mioara had for those around her.

I thank you, too. And don't forget to remember us in your prayers.

* * *

MARIA, *we've heard from your daddy that you're the "second mommy," that you help him with the household. Is it difficult to help Daddy raise your siblings?*

MARIA: Well, it's difficult to a certain extent, but I've gotten used to these responsibilities throughout the years, and I could say I can manage them—they're no longer obstacles for me. I manage, especially because I have siblings who listen to me and don't cause me any trouble. Sometimes there are conflicts, as in any family with several siblings: each one with his or her opinion, issue, desire to do things their own way, but in the end we reach a compromise, an acceptable agreement for everybody.

Do you remember an event in your life when you realized God helps and loves you?

I believe there isn't just one event; we basically feel God is always near and helps us and doesn't leave us. Although Mom is no longer here, we feel she's near us in spirit. Fr. Arsenie, our spiritual father, also tells us that, no matter what happens, Mommy is near us and we shouldn't feel alone. I feel it; I never feel abandoned. I feel her near me.

What brings you the greatest joy in life?

Well, I rejoice knowing that deep inside me there is a loving, understanding person, who helps her family. And I greatly rejoice and I'm happy, knowing I have an important role in my family. This gives me strength to move forward, seeing all my siblings happy that they have me. This makes me happy.

What do you believe was your mother's greatest virtue?

She had many.... First and foremost, she was a born fighter, and she never showed that she was not well or that she suffered. She always sought to keep us, the children, uplifted, and to support us. Although feeble, she did everything she could for us to feel that she was alive. And indeed, that's the way it was—she was the energy of the house.

Please convey a message to children who are in the same situation, having lost one of their parents, and going through difficult times.

I would tell them to not despair, because God takes care of them from above. Although it might seem hard for them in the beginning, they will see the wounds of their souls start to heal in time—slowly, slowly. And I would tell them about the happiness of their parent who has gone to the Lord, to reflect on the fact that there, up above, he or she is happy, and this has to make them happy, too. If a person is happy you should be happy, also.

What do you want to do in life?

I wish to be able to help others in need, as others have helped me. That's the mission I want to carry on. I want to help as many people as possible, and to take care of my younger brothers and sisters.

May God give you the strength to do so, and may your zeal always burn within you!

Thank you!

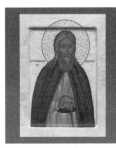 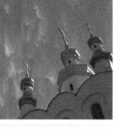

Saint Herman of Alaska Brotherhood

Since 1965, the St. Herman of Alaska Brotherhood has been publishing Orthodox Christian books and magazines.

View our catalog, featuring over fifty titles, and order online, at
www.sainthermanmonastery.com

You can also write us for a free printout of our catalog:

St. Herman of Alaska Brotherhood
P. O. Box 70
Platina, CA 96076
USA

CANCER, MY LOVE

*Text typeset in Agmena, titles in Veljovic Script. Both typefaces designed by Jovica Veljović.
Printed on fifty-five pound Glatfelter Offset paper, and notch bound at Thomson-Shore, Inc., Dexter, Michigan.*